THE LONE STAR
HIKING TRAIL

The Official Guide to the Longest Wilderness Footpath in Texas

D0963946

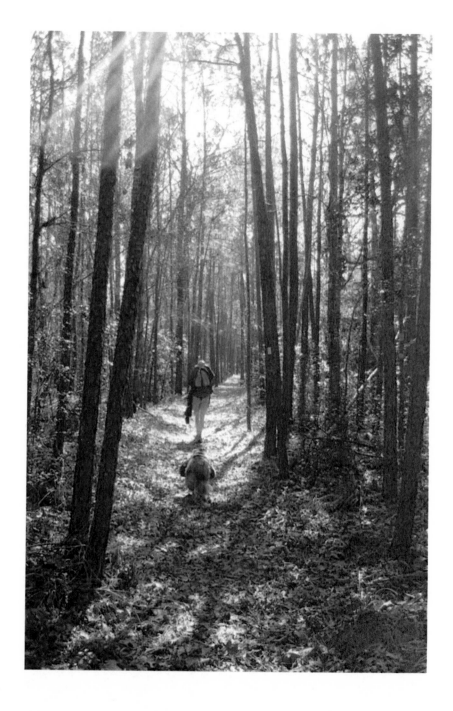

THE LONE STAR
★ HIKING TRAIL

The Official Guide to the Longest Wilderness Footpath in Texas

Karen Borski Somers

WILDERNESS PRESS . . . *on the trail since 1967*

BERKELEY, CA

The Lone Star Hiking Trail: The Official Guide to the
Longest Wilderness Footpath in Texas

1st EDITION 2009

Front cover photo copyright © 2009 by Laurence Parent Photography
Interior photos by Karen Borski Somers, except for the following: p. 5: courtesy of the
    East Texas Research Center; Steen Library, Forest History Collections, Stephen F.
    Austin State University, Nacogdoches, Texas; p. 8: courtesy of James Weatherby;
    p. 33: Poison oak and poison sumac, courtesy of Robert H. Mohlenbrock, USDA,
    and poison ivy, courtesy of Jonathan Sachs; and p. 102: courtesy of Cathy A. Murphy,
    LSHT Club
Maps: Andy Somers, Karen Borski Somers, and Scott McGrew
Cover design: Lisa Pletka
Text design: Annie Long
Book editor: Laura Shauger

ISBN 978-0-89997-504-7

Manufactured in the United States of America

Published by: **Wilderness Press**
            1345 8th Street
            Berkeley, CA 94710
            (800) 443-7227; FAX **(510) 558-1696**
            info@wildernesspress.com
            www.wildernesspress.com

Visit our website for a complete listing of our books and for ordering information.

Cover photos: Big Creek Scenic Area (*front*); Tarkington Bayou (*back*)
Frontispiece: A late winter's morning in the Big Woods Section of the Lone Star
                   Hiking Trail

SAFETY NOTICE: Although Wilderness Press and the author have made every attempt to
ensure that the information in this book is accurate at press time, they are not responsible
for any loss, damage, injury, or inconvenience that may occur to anyone while using this
book. You are responsible for your own safety and health while in the wilderness. The fact
that a trail is described in this book does not mean that it will be safe for you. Be aware
that trail conditions can change from day to day. Always check local conditions, know
your own limitations, and consult a map.

Contents

Foreword

by Marcus Woolf

I t's a strange thing to march down a trail with a measuring wheel, slowly ticking off the distance, foot by foot, watching carefully for that magic number—5280 feet (the number of feet in a mile). Time to once again hit the reset button.

Mapping a trail and simply hiking it are two very different things. Creating a guidebook requires incredible discipline and attention to detail, and this is precisely what Karen Somers brings to *The Lone Star Hiking Trail*. As she measures each step, she notes the fine details—seasonal streams, potential camping spots, and the character of the forest, from the "jungle-like" feel of a stand of dwarf palmettos to the waterfall in a "secret nook" of the trail's Magnolia Section. Accompanying her descriptive prose are helpful charts that allow hikers to quickly glance at notable waypoints that lie along the way. Karen achieves a great balance with her work, carefully weaving together crucial data and keen observations that will pique a hiker's interest. It is one thing to tell people when to turn left or right and where water sources lie; it is another to capture the sights and sounds of a place and draw the reader into the scene.

Many people take the first steps toward writing a guidebook, but soon abandon the project due to the sheer effort involved. Others enjoy a few days of hiking where they jot down the various plants, animals, and natural features along the way. And more hikers have embraced the idea of marking their routes with a GPS unit. But to do these things, and more, day after day, in blazing heat, numbing cold, or relentless downpour—this is where many book projects wither.

Having recently completed a trail guide for the Atlanta area, I can appreciate Karen's determination in mapping the 128 miles that make up the Lone Star Trail and nearby loops. The complex nature of the project—recording information with the GPS, writing notes, taking photographs, pushing that wheel—can become a weary exercise. At some point, a person's love for a place and the desire to share it become the fuel that sustains the effort. One thing I know from seeing this piece of work is that Karen has a special place in her heart for this path and the wild lands of her native Texas.

A project like this requires not only love, but practical experience. Karen has thru-hiked the 2175-mile Appalachian Trail and the 2650-mile Pacific Crest Trail. When she and her husband, Andy, trekked along the PCT, Karen published a wonderfully descriptive blog that first introduced me to her writing ability and keen eye. That five-month journey over formidable terrain honed her mapping skills and gave her the confidence to chronicle the Lone Star Trail. Under the cool blue winter skies of Texas, she often hiked with little more than the rattle of a measuring wheel to keep her company. Having experienced the same type of journey myself, I can imagine her pausing on a quiet stretch of trail and leaning over to press the reset button, watching it roll from 5280 feet to zero. With many more miles to go, I can picture her standing still for a moment to hear the winds in the pines. She wipes the sweat from her brow and smiles, remembering that this is not just work, but a chance to share something wonderful.

Marcus Woolf *has written for outdoor publications such as* Outside *and* Backpacker, *and is the senior editor at* GearTrends. *Most recently he wrote the hiking guide* Afoot & Afield Atlanta *published by Wilderness Press.*

Preface

When I thru-hiked the Lone Star Hiking Trail (LSHT) over the course of nine days in February 2006, I carried a GPS unit, pushed a measuring wheel, and took verbal notes on a tape recorder. It took time to get used to juggling all this equipment while trying to hike 100 miles, even though I had help from my friend Debbie Richardson. I followed up that first, continuous hike with shorter outings to confirm or acquire further information.

I used a Garmin 60 CS GPS unit to chart the LSHT track and, ultimately, to generate the section maps. I recorded trail mileage using a mechanical measuring wheel with an error rate of approximately +/-1 percent. Trail descriptions and observations were derived from voice notes taken on audiotape during the hike. When I sat down after that first hike to look at all the data I'd collected on the trail, I quickly realized that the really hard work had not even started.

One of my fears associated with authoring this guidebook is that, with more publicity, the LSHT may cease to be the "forgotten trail," ripe in solitude, that I love so much. But then I think about the people, like me, who have lived in southeast Texas for a long time, believing that the only long-distance hiking trails were in other states. It's these people who I hope to inspire and educate about the LSHT. They are the ones who will love it most and, ultimately, protect it.

So, what did I think about my time on the LSHT? After having hiked all over the U.S., I found everything I needed on this little trail that's been hiding in my own backyard for more than 30 years. The LSHT may not have spectacular views of mountains, and some may say that it's flat and monotonous, but I discovered a special kind of peace in the deep woods among the ancient bayous and tall pines. If you are interested in reading

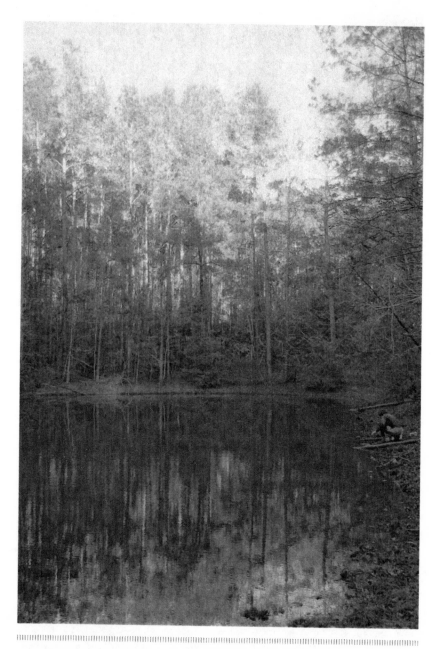

A small trailside pond in the Huntsville Section makes a picturesque setting for a camp.

more about my thru-hike, check out my online journal at **www.trailjournals. com/lonestar**.

If you want to support the LSHT, join the LSHT Club at **http://www. lshtclub.com** or the Houston Regional Group of the Sierra Club at **http:// houston.sierraclub.org**. Members of both groups volunteer their labor and funds to keep the LSHT marked, maintained, and open to hikers. They also plan group hikes, trail maintenance work hikes, and overnight outings, providing opportunities to support the LSHT and to meet others who enjoy hiking, backpacking, bird-watching, and nature.

If you come across any changes in trail conditions, resupply options, or accommodations near the trail, or if you wish to report any errors, suggestions, or comments, please contact me care of Wilderness Press at info@wildernesspress.com. I will review all submitted information for use in subsequent editions. Your help in keeping the information in this book accurate is very important and much appreciated.

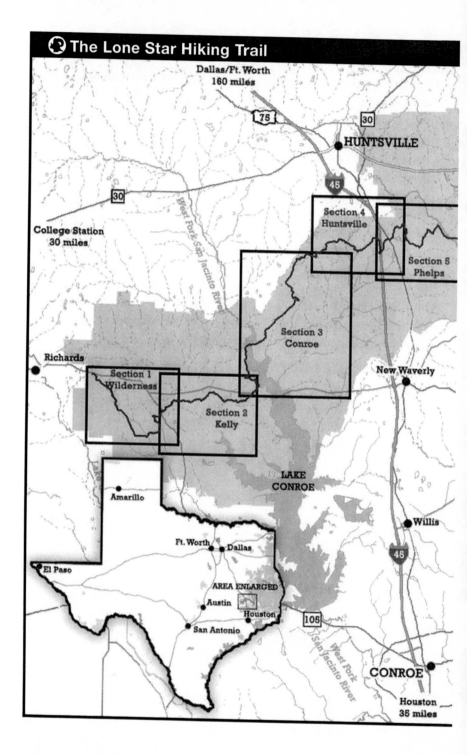

⊙ The Lone Star Hiking Trail

Dallas/Ft. Worth
160 miles

75

30

HUNTSVILLE

30

College Station
30 miles

West Fork San Jacinto River

Section 4
Huntsville

Section 5
Phelps

Section 3
Conroe

Richards

Section 1
Wilderness

New Waverly

Section 2
Kelly

LAKE
CONROE

Amarillo

Willis

45

Ft. Worth   Dallas

El Paso

AREA ENLARGED

Austin

Houston

105

San Antonio

West Fork San Jacinto River

CONROE

Houston
35 miles

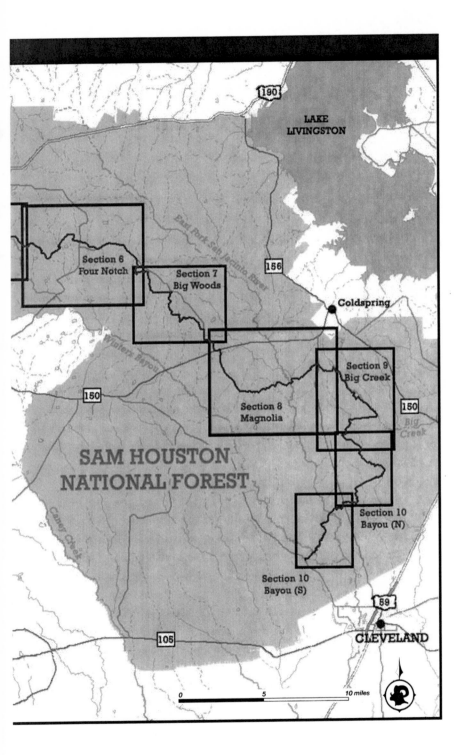

From the Lone Star Hiking Trail Club

||||||||||||||||||||||||||||||||||||||||||||||||||||||||||||||||||||||||||||||||||||||||||||||||||||||||||||||||||||||||||||||||||||||

the **Lone Star Hiking Trail** (LSHT) is a jewel set in the canopied background of a dense, exotic, semitropical forest. Occasional creek bottoms and ridges offer a changing variety of trees and other plant life. There are more than 100 miles of trails accessible year-round, and more than 30 different common wild animals, including deer, wild pigs, bobcats, and coyotes. Most of the wildlife is nocturnal, but animals are occasionally seen by dayhikers.

The LSHT is a window of opportunities for anyone interested in hiking. Friendships can be cultivated through club hikes and volunteer work on the trail is a way to serve a bigger cause. Personal hiking techniques can be honed for the Continental Divide Trail or the jungles of Central America. Navigation or nighttime hiking skills can be developed. On a more personal level, hikers can simply go out, use the trails, and recharge their batteries on the weekend to return to civilization refreshed.

The Lone Star Hiking Trail Club (LSHTC) was formed in 1995 on National Trails Day and is affiliated with the American Hiking Society. Our mission is (1) to educate the public about location, use, and needs of the hiking trails of Texas, with emphasis on the LSHT, (2) to provide volunteer assistance for trail maintenance and improvement, and (3) to maintain Internet resources that focus on information related to hiking and maintaining trails. Each year the members of the LSHTC lead over 300 hikers and trail maintenance workers on bi-weekly hikes and other activities and contribute more than 500 volunteer hours to hiker education and trail improvement.

This book is your guide to an unforgettable adventure in the Sam Houston National Forest, a cosmic wonderland of nature. Happy trails!

John S. Copenhaver
President, **Lone Star Hiking Trail Club**

A Brief History and Introduction

he story of the Lone Star Hiking Trail began in 1966 when a small group of members from the Lone Star Chapter of the Sierra Club discussed the lack of hiking trails in Texas. Orrin Bonney suggested that what was needed was a 100-mile hiking trail that would run through East Texas forests and follow old logging railroads, pipelines, and woods roads, and have places to camp every 10 miles. Other members, including Brohman Wilkin and Emil Kindschy, liked the idea and immediately began researching the feasibility. The Sierra Club approached the U.S. Forest Service, which administers the Sam Houston National Forest, through which the proposed route would run.

The Forest Service responded positively, and in 1967 work began on the trail. Much of the trail construction was done by volunteer labor, under the auspices of the Forest Service, and by 1972 most of the Lone Star Hiking Trail was completed. In 1978 the last portion of the 128-mile trail (including loop trails) was finished. My own introduction to this "nature path" began in the late 1970s as a hiker on the trail. Like my predecessors and those who will walk the Lone Star Hiking Trail far into the future, I have found delight, surprise, and solitude meandering along this shaded and secluded path.

The Lone Star Hiking Trail winds its way through shortleaf pine–post oak uplands; loblolly pine–Southern red oak–black hickory ridges and flats; white oak–Southern magnolia–loblolly pine slopes; bottomland hardwood floodplains of the East Fork of the San Jacinto River; Winters Bayou, Caney Creek, and Little Lake Creek that host water oak, American elm, water hickory, hackberry, swamp chestnut oak, green ash, and many other species of hardwood trees.

The trail offers something for hikers of every ability, from easy scenic loops that can be done in a few hours, to sections of the trail that can be hiked

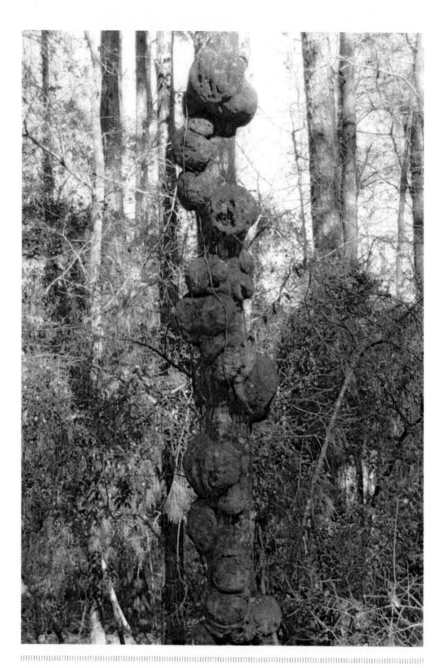

A young tree trunk covered in large galls is a strange sight along the trail in the Phelps Section.

in a day, to weeklong backpacking trips. Walking past the picturesque shores of Lake Conroe, slipping through the bottomlands of Caney Creek, camping in seclusion near Winters Bayou, kids, moms, dads, Scouts, naturalists, and the explorer and adventurer in all of us can take something from the Lone Star Hiking Trail. There are those who want to make the Lone Star Hiking Trail into something it is not; it's not for horses, bikes, or motorized vehicles, but it is for everyone with a love for wildlands, a pair of walking shoes, and the restless spirit of curiosity.

But we need to give back, too. Trail maintenance is a never-ending but joyful duty, and is always needed to ensure that this quiet, mysterious, footpath to solitude continues. Except for maintenance of bridges and signage by the Forest Service, the upkeep of the Lone Star Hiking Trail is still done by volunteers.

Some have called the Lone Star Hiking Trail the "best-kept secret in Texas." To help make it less of a secret, it has also been a long-time dream of the Sierra Club to have a guidebook for the trail. The early founders of the trail would be very pleased to see this guidebook. Come join Karen Somers and the rest of us "out on the trail." You'll be glad you did: You'll come back refreshed and your life changed. See you soon on the Lone Star Hiking Trail!

> Brandt Mannchen
> Forest Management Issue Chair
> **Lone Star Chapter of the Sierra Club**

chapter
one

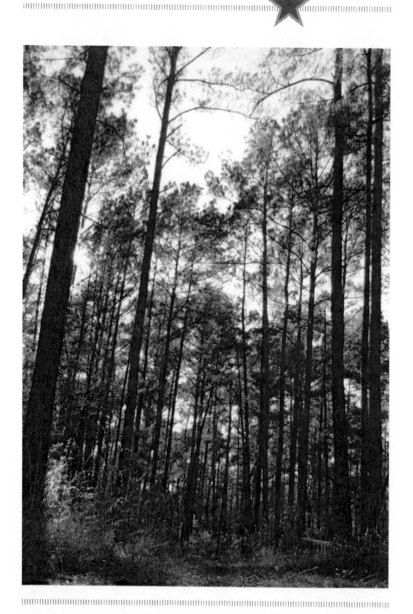

Tall pines in the Wilderness Section on the eastern end of the LSHT

history of
the trail

HIDDEN IN THE DEPTHS OF
the Sam Houston National Forest, a
little over an hour from the bustle of
downtown Houston, is a little-known
trail where one can escape for a long,
peaceful walk in the woods. This
magical retreat is the Lone Star Hiking
Trail (LSHT), a footpath that stretches
unbroken for 96 miles through the Piney
Woods of East Texas. The LSHT, part
of which is designated as a National
Recreation Trail, is limited to foot travel
and is the longest continuously marked
hiking trail in the state.

The LSHT offers hikers the chance to enjoy nature in a wilderness setting that is 70 miles north of Houston and less than a half day's drive from several other large Texas cities, including Dallas, Austin, and San Antonio. Well marked and well maintained, the trail meanders in a north-swinging arc between the small community of Richards and the town of Cleveland. Five sizeable loop trails that intersect the continuous LSHT are considered part of the trail and effectively increase its length to 128 miles. Along its course, the LSHT passes through, or near, Little Lake Creek Wilderness, Lake Conroe, Stubblefield Lake, spring-fed Double Lake, Big Creek Scenic Area, and the upper wild stretches of the East Fork of the San Jacinto River.

A seemingly endless succession and variation of forests provide a paradise for tree lovers and bird-watchers. Clear-flowing sandy-bottomed creeks, hardwood wetlands, and muddy bayous cut through gently rolling forests of pine, oak, and mixed hardwood in part of Texas's famed Big Thicket. What the LSHT lacks in wide-open views, it more than makes up for in rich, diverse woodlands and peaceful solitude. It is one of the hidden jewels of Texas. To enjoy the trail it is important to know a little about it—when to hike, how to get there, and what to expect. This guidebook is intended for hikers who want to explore the LSHT for any length of time or distance.

Like many of America's long-distance trails, the LSHT remains largely a volunteer effort. Every year, hundreds of hours of labor are required to keep the trail clear of the very forest through which it passes. Clearing brush and fallen trees, building and repairing bridges and repairing and replacing trail markers constitute a nonstop job undertaken primarily by volunteers from the Lone Star Hiking Trail Club, the Houston Regional Group of the Sierra Club, and the Boy Scouts of America. These organizations need ongoing funding and volunteers. As you explore the LSHT, consider becoming a trail steward by supporting these organizations or by joining a volunteer trail work crew.

Human History of the LSHT

Native Americans

The native inhabitants of southeast Texas were seminomadic hunter-gatherers, moving seasonally in search of food. During winter, they would settle in camps, or semipermanent villages, to hunt small game, deer, bears, and buffalo. In warmer months, they moved around in search of nuts, berries, fish, and roots, sometimes trading with other Native American tribes. Some tribes also cultivated maize. Archaeological evidence indicates that Native Americans inhabited what is now the Sam Houston National Forest as far back as 7,000 years ago.

The Hasinai Caddo, an offshoot tribe of the great mound-building civilization centered in the Mississippi River valley, resided between the Neches and Sabine Rivers. Because of their strong cultural roots and inland location, they tended to settle into small villages where they practiced agriculture and developed artistic clothing, wood carvings, and ceramics. The Karankawa lived nearer to the coast in small family groups, often traveling in search of food. The coastal-based subsistence living of the Karankawa, along with their unique language, kept them separate from many inland tribes. The Atapakan-speaking tribes—the Patiri, Bidai, Deadose, and Akokisa (also spelled Orcoquisac)—lived and roamed throughout the Trinity and San Jacinto River valleys. All of these groups converged on the Big Thicket region for hunting forays and engaged in a long-distance trade network. East Texas seashells and deer skins could be traded for the furs of the northern pine marten or clay pottery from the desert southwest.

The Atapakan tribes and Karankawa succumbed to diseases introduced by early European explorers and settlers. By the mid-1800s, nearly all of the native inhabitants of southeast Texas had vanished. Only vague accounts of their cultures remain today. Some East Texas Caddo survived disease only to be driven from their native lands by the Europeans, eventually settling in Oklahoma in 1859 (where their descendants live today).

Early European Explorers

Álvar Núñez Cabeza de Vaca, a Spanish conquistador, was shipwrecked on Galveston Island on the southeast Texas coast in November 1528. Over the next four years, he lived with the Native Americans of East Texas, becoming a trader and medicine man, and eventually walking thousands of miles through what is now the southwestern U.S. to Spanish outposts in Mexico. He eventually returned to Europe and published an important account of his remarkable journey through the unknown region. By the time other explorers ventured into this area, almost a century later, many of the native inhabitants had already vanished, victims of disease and war. Cabeza de Vaca's account is a glimpse of East Texas before European colonization irrevocably changed the land, culture, and ecology.

The French explorer René-Robert Cavalier, Sieur de La Salle, journeyed into southeast Texas in 1687 after France laid claim to the lands of the Mississippi watershed. La Salle planned to establish outposts as he ventured northward up the Mississippi River, but he was murdered in a mutiny near Navasota, Texas, before he was able to carry out his expedition. A few years later, in 1690, the first East Texas mission was built by the Spanish for the Caddo near the settlement of Nacogdoches, an effort by Spain to gain control over the region. French influence eventually succumbed to the Spanish presence, although the French continued active trade with the Akokisa and Bidai. Eventually, in 1823, the first American pioneers settled in East Texas as part of Stephen Austin's original colony. American pioneers and frontierspeople continued to trickle into the state; they eventually formed a small militia that revolted against Mexico and won independence for Texas in 1836. As the country of Texas transitioned to U.S. statehood in 1845, the newly arrived European residents of East Texas had already settled into the land—farming, logging, and ranching.

Logging and the Timber Industry

The logging boom peaked in East Texas starting in the 1880s and spurred the development of hundreds of mill towns. With the forests of the northern and eastern U.S. already harvested, investors and lumberjacks flocked to the huge expanse of untapped virgin forest that covered the gently rolling lands of East Texas. By the 1920s, 18 million acres of the East

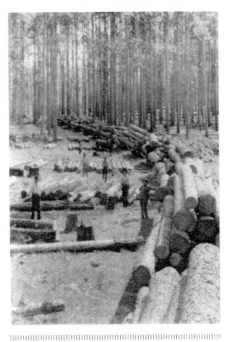

The original longleaf pines of East Texas were clear-cut and railed to mills at the turn of the century.

Texas Piney Woods had been cut, yielding an astounding 59 billion board feet of lumber.

Most of the mill towns and railroads that had sprung up overnight during the logging boom were quickly abandoned when the forests became depleted. The land left behind was no longer a rich, thick old-growth forest. Most of it had been cut to the ground and abandoned. The lumber companies either went bankrupt or moved westward in search of more timber. (Some of the old logging railroad beds from this era are still visible in the woods along the LSHT; in fact, the trail is actually routed on a few of them.) In 1934, the U.S. government authorized the purchase of some of the unwanted, depleted lands in East Texas, creating the Sabine, Angelina, Davy Crockett, and Sam Houston national forests. Over the next 80 years, the U.S. Forest Service (USFS) managed the replanting and harvesting of these lands.

Sam Houston National Forest

The 163,037-acre Sam Houston National Forest is contained within three Texas counties: Montgomery, San Jacinto, and Walker. The USFS is responsible for soil conservation, natural resources, and sustainable use practices within the national forests. Their multiple-use management policy means that logging, hunting, fishing, mining, drilling, off-road vehicle use, hiking, and camping are all allowed within national forest boundaries, as long as they meet the regulations of the USFS. Generally, the LSHT is routed well away from heavily used areas of the forest, but hikers should be aware that they may encounter these activities. Although much of the Sam Houston National Forest is an unbroken woodland expanse, there are many private landholdings within the national forest, some of which force the LSHT to follow roads. Road walks can follow anything from an old dirt road to a few paved highways, taking hikers past farms, cemeteries, churches, and even contemporary neighborhoods.

Creation of the Lone Star Hiking Trail

The LSHT was conceived during a backpacking trip when a small group of Sierra Club members were camping in the Sam Houston National Forest in 1966. Lamenting that there weren't many hiking trails in the region, the hikers decided to approach the USFS to gain permission to plan and build a trail that would traverse the length of the national forest. With logistical and financial assistance from the Sierra Club and Shell Oil Company, volunteers began construction in 1967 and completed the LSHT by 1972. Long-term oversight of the trail was turned over to the USFS, but

Markers found along the eastern 28 miles of the LSHT indicate National Recreation Trail status.

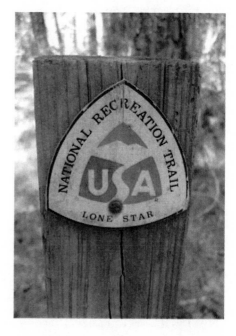

volunteers continued to maintain the trail and spent time in the late 1970s expanding the trail to its current length. Today, the LSHT is supported by the Lone Star Hiking Trail Club and the Houston Regional Group of the Sierra Club, which organizes volunteer maintenance efforts and oversees trail issues. Volunteers from the Boy Scouts of America, also labor to keep the trail marked, bridged, and cleared.

The National Trail System Act of 1968 set the framework for the LSHT to receive federal protection; however, only the eastern 28 miles of the LSHT have been designated as a National Recreation Trail to date. Despite overarching regulations stating that the entire LSHT is off-limits to motorized vehicles, stock animals, wagons, and bicycles, it continues to be threatened by misuse and neglect. Its "footpath only" designation is shared by only a few other trails in the U.S., but like many of these other trails, the LSHT continues to battle pressure from outside interests that would damage or destroy it. Without a protective buffer, other activities and interests within the national forest can damage the trail (examples include logging, road-building, drilling, and fire control activities). Additionally, others want the trail opened up for use by horseback riders and mountain bikers. The Sierra Club continues to lead a long-term fight for a protective buffer on either side of the trail, as well as an ongoing battle to maintain the LSHT's unique status as a trail preserved for foot travel only.

Natural History of the LSHT

Geology

During the Paleozoic Era, about 500 million years ago, the edge of the ancient North American continent began to rift along its southern edge. As the land subsided, a shallow inland sea formed, covering all of what is now East Texas. Subsequent periods of continental extension and compression formed basins in which thick deposits of marine salt were covered by sands and sediments, eventually forming significant oil and natural gas deposits. Later, river systems, such as the Trinity, Sabine, and Neches in East Texas, distributed more sediment on the coastal plains as they drained toward the Gulf of Mexico. The soils of East Texas are deep and rich; they are typically light-colored acidic sands, sandy loam mixed with deposits of clay (or clay-shale) and occasional mineral-rich red soils.

Plant Life

The LSHT's western terminus lies at the very edge of the great eastern deciduous forest of North America. West of the town of Richards, the land transitions from the thick Piney Woods to more open post-oak savannah

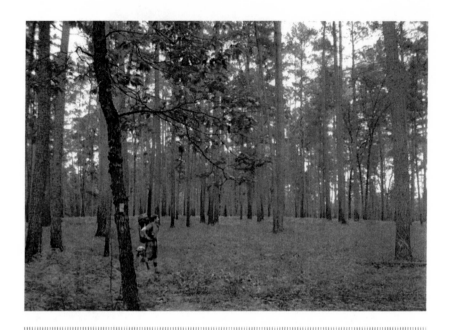

A hiker and his canine companion pause to admire the trunks of mature pines blackened by a recent prescribed burn.

and blackland prairie. Along this meeting of major biogeographic regions, complex woodlands have evolved. At first glance, the untrained eye may only see forests dominated by loblolly and shortleaf pines. Look a little closer and discover a unique mix of species. The Sam Houston National Forest is the westernmost range of many eastern trees (such as white oak, longleaf pine, and Southern magnolia) and also home to plants that originated in drier western climates (such as prickly pear cacti and yucca). The diverse plant mosaic in this region can also be traced to the last ice age, when species from other parts of the continent moved southward.

The large terrestrial ecological region called the Piney Woods stretches across most of East Texas and into parts of Arkansas, Louisiana, and Oklahoma. The Piney Woods are dominated by several species of pine, as well as being home to a large variety of hardwood tree species. The Piney Woods are not an unbroken homogeneous woodland but consist of a tapestry of interwoven ecological environments, each supporting different species.

While hiking on the LSHT, you will see only some of the ecosystems that compose the Piney Woods and the nearby subregion called the Big Thicket, an extremely biodiverse area that contains one of the highest species counts for an area of its size in the U.S. (Unfortunately, only the most remote, central part of the original Big Thicket has been fully protected as a national preserve near the eastern end of the LSHT.)

Many of the region's ecological zones are easy to identify, while others may require more study using a tree guide. A few of the most common ecosystems by tree type are as follows: bottomlands composed of oak, hickory, sycamore, ash, sweetgum, alder, river birch, black willow, and maple; swamps composed of bald cypress, swamp tupelo, water hickory, and water elm; seasonally inundated flats composed of dwarf palmettos growing among a mix of hardwood trees; sloping, well-drained land comprised of American beech, Southern magnolia, and white oak; and, finally, pure stands of loblolly and shortleaf pine. A rich variety of mosses, grasses, ferns, mushrooms, and wildflowers prospers beneath the canopy of the forest. Wildflower enthusiasts can spot spring beauty, rose vervain, and Halbert-leaf rose-mallow, as well as wild orchids and sundews.

The nature of this great forest is changing; today there is more pine in proportion to hardwood. After the first wave of commercial logging denuded much of the area by the early 1900s, the fast-growing slash pine was widely planted throughout East Texas. Meanwhile, diverse bottomland ecosystems were destroyed by the creation of reservoirs. Fire was once a regular and natural force that had an integral effect on the composition of the forests, but due to human intervention, fire has been widely suppressed. The resulting monoculture pine plantations support more disease and destructive pests, such as the pine bark beetle. While the USFS has become a better steward of its lands, often prescribing burns to mimic natural conditions, it has also allowed extensive pine plantations to continue to exist in support of the timber industry.

Virtually no virgin forest remains in East Texas. During the 1970s and '80s, after the forests had somewhat recovered from their initial exploitation, clear-cutting of the forest again drastically increased. This process, along with the clearing of land for development and agriculture, has destroyed well over half of the original 5,000 square miles of habitat in East Texas that once harbored the greatest diversity of plant and wildlife in North America. However, hikers walking on the LSHT can still see enormous pines growing in parklike settings (the native loblolly pine reached six feet in diameter and up to 170 feet in height, though most nowadays are only half that size), miles of mature magnolias and beech, and extensive palmetto swamps. Some of these trees are more than 100 years old. Yet, they merely hint at what this great forest used to be. Where they are given lasting protection, East Texas's woods will continue to evolve into more complex and mature habitats resembling their former grandeur.

Animal Life

Once, East Texas was home to cougars, wolves, black bears, and jaguars. As Europeans began to settle the land, hunting and habitat loss took their toll, and all of these large predators gradually disappeared. Red wolves, smaller cousins to the gray wolf, were able to hang on until 1990, when the last wild individuals were trapped and removed to be placed in a captive breeding project. Coyotes and bobcats prosper and are now the largest predators remaining in East Texas. Sporadic sightings of mountain lions and black bears in East Texas have been on the rise, but it is still believed that no breeding populations have been established.

Some of the species that have returned from the brink of extinction in East Texas include the river otter, beaver, bald eagle, and American alligator. Common white-tailed deer and eastern wild turkey were hunted to the point of eradication in the early 1900s and recovered only after reintroduction programs proved successful in the mid- to late 20th century. Bison were not as fortunate; their numbers never recovered in Texas as they did in a few other areas of the U.S. Even today, there are mammals that face extinction in East Texas, such as the Plains spotted skunk and two species of bats. Less visible endangered aquatic species found in the larger waterways of the region include the paddlefish and American eel, both of which have suffered due to reservoir construction.

Common mammals of East Texas include many well-known species of the southeastern deciduous forest, such as the raccoon, Eastern fox squirrel, gray squirrel, and opossum. A beaverlike rodent called the nutria and domestic pigs are both animals that were released or escaped into the wild from farms and have prospered at the expense of native species. The nine-banded armadillo migrated on its own northward from Mexico to the southeastern U.S. and is the animal most likely to be seen or heard by campers. Many types of snakes and turtles, as well as amphibians, fish, and an amazing variety of insects, also inhabit the Piney Woods.

Texas is regarded as a bird-watcher's paradise. In addition to year-long resident birds, the mild winters of the Texas Gulf Coast offer winter refuge to scores of migratory bird species, such as the Arctic peregrine falcon. The rich and varied forest ecology of East Texas provides many differing bird habitats within a small area. Thick Piney Woods are home to the resident pine warbler, brown-headed nuthatch, barred owl, and summer tanager. Bottomlands harbor the pileated woodpecker, Carolina chickadee, and Kentucky warbler. Swamps and bayous provide homes for Swainson's warblers, wood ducks, and fish crows. Reservoirs, like Lake Conroe, have attracted bald eagles spending the winter in the warm climate of East Texas.

Due to the conversion of much of the native longleaf pine–oak–palmetto forests of East Texas to pine plantation, cropland, and reservoir, many bird populations have diminished. Probably the most well-known rare bird that lives year-round in the Sam Houston National Forest is the red-cockaded woodpecker, a species that was declared endangered in 1970 and has been steadily declining over the last 15 years. These small, cardinal-sized woodpeckers are frequently spotted by observant hikers, especially near Stubblefield Lake. They require parklike stands of mature native pine trees in which they build nesting cavities, a habitat now being protected for these birds. The red-cockaded woodpecker has a distinctive large white cheek patch (males have a small red spot behind their eyes that give the species its name). Its unique high-pitched, squeaky call can be recognized at considerable distances.

chapter two

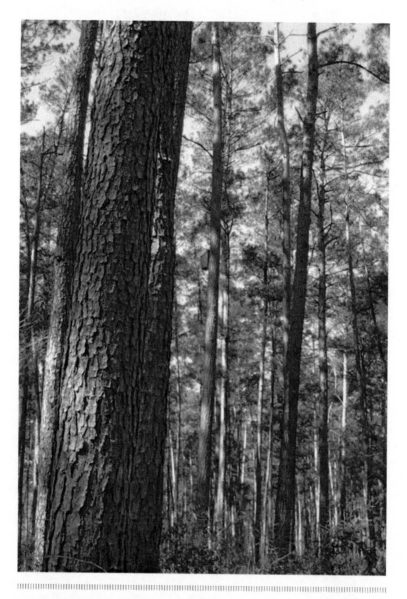

A wood box (upper center of photo) provides shelter for birds and
bats high in a pine in the Kelly Section.

hiking
the trail

HIKES ON THE LSHT CAN RANGE
from short strolls to multiday backpacking trips. Every year, a few hikers even opt to thru-hike the LSHT, walking the whole trail in one continuous journey. Hikers enjoy a well-marked, nearly level trail, broken only by a few country road walks and abounding in backcountry camping opportunities. Loops along the LSHT add another 32 miles of trail to the continuous 96-mile footpath.

How to Use This Book

This guidebook focuses on the main, continuous LSHT footpath. Side trails that intersect the LSHT are noted and shown on maps but not described in detail.

For organizational purposes, the LSHT is broken into 10 sections, each roughly the length of a long dayhike. Section boundaries are defined by road crossings or access points. Each section includes an overview; information on trail access, parking, water availability, access to supplies, and accommodations; a detailed trail description; a chart of GPS coordinates for major trail features; a mileage chart summarizing trail features by distance from west to east (and vice versa); and a trail map. For reference, the mileage charts are consolidated in Appendix D (page 162).

There is no right or wrong direction to hike the LSHT. This guide contains trail descriptions written from west to east only because one direction had to be chosen for the guide and established mile markers already line the trail increasing in order from west to east. *Westbound hikers (those hiking from east to west) will have to mentally reverse the trail descriptions, changing "left" to "right" and vice versa, as well as reading the trail descriptions "backward."*

GPS coordinates (using Datum WGS84) are listed for trailheads and major trail features. Mileage chart notes abbreviations are as follows:

MILEAGE CHART KEY

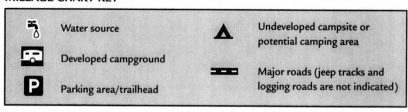

🚰	Water source	▲	Undeveloped campsite or potential camping area
🚐	Developed campground		
🅿	Parking area/trailhead	▬▬	Major roads (jeep tracks and logging roads are not indicated)

Maps

The USFS publishes a map of the entire Sam Houston National Forest that shows the route of the LSHT (see Appendix A, page 157, for information on ordering maps). It does not show as much detail as the maps in this guide but does provide a good overview of the area and road system surrounding the LSHT.

The detailed section maps in this book are derived from USGS 7.5-minute quadrangle maps. On each map, the LSHT is indicated by a solid line. Dashed lines show side trails that intersect the LSHT and indicate the previous and/or next sections of the LSHT. As a general rule, larger roads are denoted by a heavier black line. Small roads (jeep tracks and logging roads) appear as unlabeled, dashed

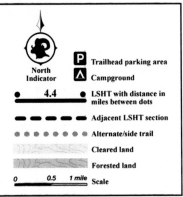

lines. Pipelines are dashed lines and are typically labeled. Major water features are shaded gray. *Not every shaded water feature offers hikers a viable water source—many creeks in the area are dry most of the year. Use each section's trail description and mileage chart to plan your water sources.* At the time of this printing, magnetic declination is approximately 3.5 degrees east along the entire length of the LSHT.

Trail and Mile Markers

The LSHT is a continuously marked footpath, meaning that a hiker walking in either direction should be able to see trail markers indicating the pathway at regular intervals, usually one marker being within sight of the next. In addition to regular trail markers, nearly every mile of the LSHT is also marked and labeled.

LSHT *trail markers* are 2- x 4-inch unpainted aluminum plates that have been nailed to trees, posts, or poles at eye level adjacent to the trail. Double sets of markers, or tilted markers, indicate turns, trail junctions, or places where hikers should pay particular attention to the route. Three markers placed together indicate one of the several designated primitive backcountry camping areas along the LSHT. A marker with a white stripe at its midsection indicates a junction of the main LSHT with a loop trail. Other intersecting trails are marked with colored paint or striped metal markers. Old-style LSHT markers were 3-inch metal triangles and may still exist along some parts of the trail.

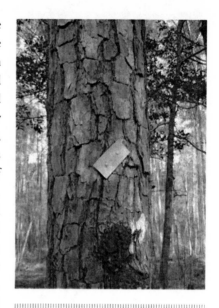

A slanted LSHT trail marker indicating a right turn ahead

Generally, the LSHT is well marked and easy to follow; however, there may be spots where trail markers are missing or infrequent (treefall and vandalism are the biggest culprits). When small sections of the trail become overgrown with brush or covered with fallen leaves, look up and scan ahead for markers. If you've been walking for more than five minutes and haven't seen a trail marker, you may have wandered off the LSHT. Turn around and retrace your steps back to the last place you saw a marker. Keep in mind that markers are often absent where the LSHT follows roads—this guide includes detailed directions to help you navigate road walks.

LSHT *mile markers* are diamond-shaped red-and-white metal tags used to indicate each of the 96 miles of the LSHT. Mile markers are usually placed on trees just above eye level, but some are also marked with a plastic post planted in the ground. A few miles do not appear to be marked, particularly on road walks, but mile markers can be easy to overlook while you are walking and watching the trail in front of you. The mile markers are accurate, except where noted in the trail description. In a few sections, old wooden posts with miles marked upon their tops stand along the trail; all of these are outdated and inaccurate.

Trail Access and Parking

There are plenty of regular LSHT trailhead access points where free parking is available. These trailhead parking areas are described and mapped in each section. The Forest Service reports a very low incidence of trailhead vandalism, but it is always advisable to lock valuables out of sight or in the trunk of your car. If you plan to park your car at Stubblefield Lake Campground, Huntsville State Park, or Double Lake Recreation Area, expect to notify park personnel of your plans and to pay entrance fees. Each of these parks also has nearby LSHT trailhead parking areas that do not require a fee.

Trail Conditions

The LSHT meanders through flat to gently rolling forests of varying age and type. Altitude on the LSHT is roughly between 150 and 400 feet above sea level. The hiker never ascends more than 75 feet at one time; these climbs are extremely gentle. Creeks represent the most difficult natural features to cross on the LSHT. Large creeks, rivers, and extensive wetlands are bridged, although bridges may occasionally be destroyed during floods. Most creeks along the trail are usually dry or contain water only a few inches deep—though some have cut V-shaped ravines up to eight feet deep that require short, steep scrambles down and up the banks.

The LSHT traverses a broad range of soil conditions, from well-drained sandy uplands to incessantly muddy bottomlands. Hikers should not have serious difficulty negotiating muddy areas, but should expect soggy footwear on occasion. Potentially problematic areas are noted in the trail descriptions. You may encounter blowdown (fallen trees lying across the trail) and overgrown trail, but these are usually not persistent obstacles. Trail conditions are always subject to change, particularly after big storms. Check with the Sam Houston National Forest District Office or the Lone Star Hiking Trail Club for the latest LSHT conditions.

Seasons and Weather

IIIIIIIIIIIIIIIIIIIIIIIIIIIIIIIIIIIIIIIIIIIIIIIIIIIIIIIIIIIIIIIIIIIIIIIIIIIIIIIIIIIIIIIIIIIIIIIIIIIIIIIIIIIIIIIIIIIIIIIIIIIIIIIIIIIIIIIIIIIIIIIIIIIIIIIIIII

Biting insects, extreme heat, and fewer on-trail water sources, make hiking during the long East Texas summers challenging. From May through September, temperatures can reach the upper 90s, with high humidity levels that make the temperature feel well into the triple digits. If you venture onto the trail during these months, be prepared to hike at a slower pace, as well as to protect yourself from insects. Be aware that water sources listed in this guidebook may dry up during the hottest months.

The best seasons for hiking on the LSHT are late fall, winter, and early spring. Fall is characterized by temperature variations that are caused by intermittent cold fronts passing southeastward through the region. Cold fronts can be slow- or fast-moving and bring rain followed by rapidly falling temperatures. Winter in East Texas is generally mild, but freezing temperatures are possible. The Sam Houston National Forest receives 45 inches of rainfall per year on average. More rain falls in the spring and fall, but there is not a strict pattern. Droughts or periods of heavy rain can happen any time of year.

Tornadoes are most common in the spring, but can also occur in summer and fall. Hurricanes give more warning of their approach. Don't

TEMPERATURE RANGES ON THE TRAIL				
MONTH	AVERAGE HIGH	AVERAGE LOW	RECORD HIGH	RECORD LOW
JAN	58° F	39° F	88° F	7° F
FEB	63° F	43° F	94° F	7° F
MAR	71° F	50° F	91° F	18° F
APR	78° F	56° F	97° F	31° F
MAY	84° F	64° F	98° F	42° F
JUN	90° F	70° F	106° F	54° F
JUL	94° F	72° F	107° F	56° F
AUG	94° F	72° F	107° F	56° F
SEPT	88° F	67° F	104° F	41° F
OCT	79° F	58° F	98° F	28° F
NOV	69° F	49° F	90° F	19° F
DEC	60° F	41° F	85° F	2° F

venture onto the LSHT if a hurricane is moving toward the Texas Gulf Coast and keep a close watch on the weather during the peak of hurricane season (August and September). Although the trail is located well inland, a hurricane's high winds will reach the LSHT and can spawn tornadoes. Falling limbs and trees are common in windy conditions. Creeks and rivers can quickly rise out of their banks during heavy rain.

The following is a month-by-month guide of what to expect on the trail. Average and record temperatures are found in the chart on the opposite page.

January is one of the best months to be out on the trail. Deer hunting season ends early in the month. Daytime temperatures can range from warm to cool. Expect cool nights with temperatures below freezing on the coldest nights.

February is an excellent month to be out on the LSHT. As in January, be prepared for nighttime temperatures in the 30s and 40s with some rare nights in the 20s. Carry warm clothes but keep a T-shirt on hand for warmer days.

Ankle-deep water on the LSHT after heavy rainfall

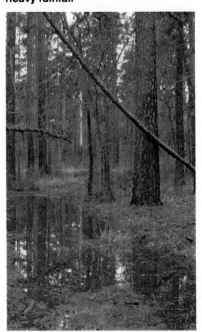

March is when the trees and bugs begin to come to life again, but it's still a great time to be in the woods. Leaves begin to unfurl, honeysuckle blooms, and birds are active. Expect a few flies and mosquitoes, but mostly enjoy the butterflies. Cold nights are possible, but rare.

April is the month of Texas's famous wildflowers. The woods have fewer flowers than the roadsides, but woodland wildflowers are unique treasures compared to their cultivated roadside cousins. Temperatures are still pleasant enough to enjoy hiking before it really warms up.

May is the wettest month of the year on average. Hiking in May is a toss-up, depending on the weather and your tolerance for heat and insects. Some days are dry and beautiful, but others are a prelude to summer.

June is the first full month of summer. Flies, ticks, spiders, mosquitoes, and chiggers make their debut, so carry insect repellent or wear long pants. Carry plenty of water and don't overexert yourself.

July and **August** are terribly hot and humid. All seasonal creeks will be dry except after heavy rains. Consider sitting these months out from hiking or take shorter hikes in the cooler hours of the day. Don't forget insect protection!

September continues to demonstrate the brutal heat of East Texas summers, but every once in a while, a minor cool front can arrive early and provide a few cooler, less humid days. Bugs continue to be an issue.

October is when both hiking and deer hunting season begin. Wear fluorescent orange hunter safety gear in the woods. Ticks are active, but you should see fewer flies and mosquitoes.

November brings increasingly better temperatures for hiking, but deer hunting season spans the entire month. Wear hunter safety colors. Bugs diminish.

December is a good time of the year to hike, except for the continuing concern about deer hunting season. Leaves fall off of deciduous trees.

Water

Access to water on the trail is primarily a concern of overnight hikers. Lack of water can be a very serious issue on the LSHT. Each section includes a general overview of water sources along the trail, as well as the detailed mileage chart listing places where water was found when I scouted the trail. These sources are noted with a 🚰 in the mileage charts; careful effort has been made to subjectively describe the type and quality of water found. Seasonal creeks are listed as "seasonal drainages." After rains, they may appear to be lush, flowing creeks, but in fact, they are dry most of the year and unreliable as water sources. Even though every effort was made to record only sources that appeared to be dependable, *it is possible that water sources listed in this book will be dry in the future.* Always carry more water than you think you'll need, in case an expected water source is dry. A general rule of thumb is that each hiker needs a minimum of three quarts of water per day in *cool* weather (that does not include water for cooking). In hot weather, carry at least one liter of drinking water for every 3 miles.

All natural water found along the LSHT should be filtered or chemically treated to prevent illness from waterborne parasites or bacteria. Even clear, clean-looking water can harbor microscopic organisms, like *Giardia lamblia*. Potable drinking water is only available near the LSHT from taps at Stubblefield Lake Campground, Huntsville State Park, and Double Lake Recreation Area.

Rules and Regulations

The LSHT is contained mostly within the Sam Houston National Forest. The rules that govern hikers on the LSHT are mostly the same as those that govern any person in the national forest. The big exception is that *horses, bicycles,*

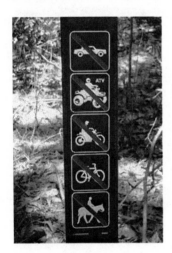

motorized vehicles, and equipment of any kind are prohibited on the LSHT. Only foot travel is allowed. Permits are not required to hike on the trail or park in LSHT trailhead parking lots. However, fees are usually required if you choose to park or camp in nearby developed campgrounds or state parks. Dogs are permitted on the LSHT, but rules require that they be leashed and under the owner's control at all times. Remember that damaging or removing any natural feature or historical or archaeological artifact or site is strictly prohibited within the national forest.

Camping

Hikers are allowed to camp anywhere along the LSHT within the national forest with a few exceptions. The LSHT traverses one specially protected area where camping is prohibited: the Big Creek Scenic Area in Section 9. Additionally, camping is not allowed inside—or within 300 feet—of any trailhead parking area. During deer rifle hunting season, the rules state

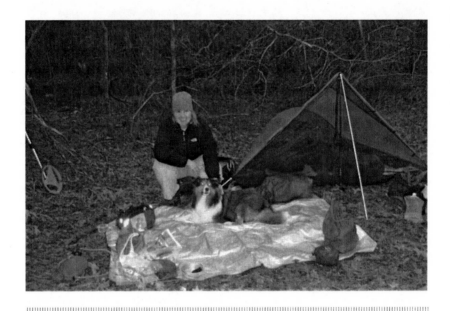

The author in camp with her dog, Buddy, in the Huntsville Section

that everyone in the national forest must camp in developed, or designated, hunter campsites. Therefore, if you plan to camp in the forest between November 1 and January 1, the Sam Houston National Forest District Office can provide advice and direction on where it is legal to camp.

The LSHT often crosses or skirts private property. Use your trail descriptions, maps, and common sense to avoid camping on private property. Disturbing or entering private property is illegal and will only diminish local support for the LSHT.

Campfires are allowed but should be built only within existing fire rings. During dry seasons, campfires may be completely banned along the LSHT. Check with the Sam Houston National Forest District Office for any restrictions on open fires before you plan to make a campfire within the woods. These restrictions are put in place to protect both you and the forest from an out-of-control wildfire. (Backpacking stoves are typically, but not always, allowed during fire bans.) Anyone responsible for causing a wildfire is also responsible for all costs of fighting that fire; the Forest Service has been increasingly vigorous in prosecuting those linked to starting forest fires.

Hunting

Hunting is allowed throughout the Sam Houston National Forest and on private property located adjacent to, and within, the boundaries of the forest. The only exception to this rule along the LSHT, is that hunting is not allowed within the Big Creek Scenic Area. Deer hunting season varies each year, but rifle season generally extends from November 1 to January 1 (the dates when camping restrictions are in effect). Bow season for deer roughly spans the month of October. Squirrel hunting season extends into February. Turkey hunting season is in the spring, typically in April. Thus, be aware that other types of hunting seasons are underway at various times during the year. Hikers are advised to wear highly visible clothing, such as fluorescent orange, during deer season.

Trail Ethics

We are only visitors in the wilderness. Preserving our wild lands requires that all who visit them use common sense and courtesy to ensure that no harm comes to them. Armed with a bit of knowledge and forethought, we can go into the woods, enjoy our trails and forests, and leave them pristine for those who follow. Before venturing out on the trail, refresh yourself on outdoor ethics.

Leave no trace means that we must leave the woods in the same condition as, if not better than, when we arrived with absolutely no trace of our passing. Small but harmful practices can accumulate over time so that what is only a trace of our passing today can become a destructive and ugly legacy as others follow in our path in the future.

Stay on the trail even in muddy spots—walking around wet areas just widens the trail into an ugly mud pit. In places, the LSHT is routed adjacent to private property. Don't jump fences, camp in fields, or otherwise trespass onto private land. Be courteous so that local landowners will continue to allow the trail to pass across their property.

Fires may be illegal and are extremely dangerous during dry seasons. Cook your backcountry meals using a backpacking stove—they are light, economical, and easy to use. Campfires should be started only within existing fire rings. Don't cut live trees or branches; use only small downed pieces of wood. Always ensure that your campfire is completely extinguished.

Camp in previously used or established sites or in areas clear of vegetation and out of sight of the trail. If you must set up in a new unused spot, be sure you are at least 200 feet away from the trail and at least 500 feet away from water sources. If every hiker created a new tent site and fire ring, the trail would cease to feel like a backcountry experience.

Wildlife should be discouraged from visiting your camp and should not suffer any harm from your visit. Always keep a clean camp and hang your food in trees away from easy access by raccoons. Never harm animals or allow your dog to chase wildlife.

Human waste should be buried four to six inches deep at least 100 feet away from the trail and at least 200 feet from creeks, rivers, or lakes. Pack used toilet paper out in ziploc bags to ease the impact of human waste along the trail.

Litter is anything that you brought into the woods. If you make the effort to pack something into the woods, then you are responsible for packing it out. Remember that fruit peelings, toilet paper, and cigarette butts take many years to degrade, and fire pits are not trash cans. It's a good practice to pick up any litter that you see, even if it's not yours.

Water is a precious resource and home to many fish and invertebrates. Don't put *anything* into any water source, even so-called biodegradable soap. Keep all bathroom activities far away from creeks, rivers, and lakes. Remember that you live downstream and may drink this water, too.

Dogs face more dangers and difficulties on the trail than humans. Ticks, chiggers, extreme heat, wildlife, and hunters all threaten dogs' health and safety. Dogs can get into skirmishes with the wild residents of the forest. Keep dogs leashed and under your direct control on the trail and in camp. Provide plenty of water and watch for signs of overexertion and heat stress.

Groups should be limited to six people or fewer. Larger groups greatly increase the possibility of damage to the trail and decrease the solitude,

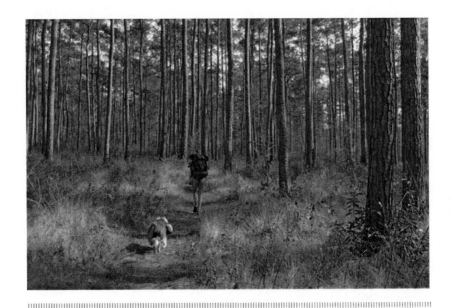

A backpacker and dog walk near Tarkington Bayou on their LSHT thru-hike.

peace, and unique experience of being in the backcountry for both the group and other hikers they encounter.

Be quiet and considerate while you are hiking and in camp. Other people visit the backcountry to get away from the noise and bustle of city life. Don't use cell phones or other noise-generating technology near other people.

If in doubt, follow the hikers' golden rule: Take only pictures, leave only footprints.

Thru-Hiking

Every year a few hikers set out to walk the entire length of the LSHT. Some hikers will piece together sections of trail over time, perhaps even dayhiking all of the LSHT. Thru-hikers are generally regarded as those who attempt a continuous, self-supported hike of the entire trail. Most thru-hikers will carry a loaded backpack and restock their food supplies somewhere along the way.

It is possible for an experienced, fit backpacker to thru-hike the LSHT without resupply in as little as four or five days. Most thru-hikers will walk at a pace that allows them to complete the trail in eight to ten days, and they will need to resupply about midway through their trek. Carrying enough food to thru-hike the entire LSHT is possible, but not recommended. Food is heavy!

There are no resupply facilities directly along the LSHT's path, but there are a few options within walking distance of the trail and many more within a short drive from the trail. Each section provides directions and distances to all potential resupply options, in addition to other amenities such as vending machines, pay phones, and hot showers.

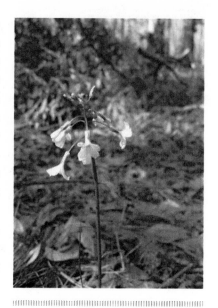

The native spring cress is a member of the mustard family and can be found along the bottomlands of Winters Bayou.

Equipment

Selection of hiking equipment is a subjective process that depends on personal experience and preference. However, there are some basic items that no one should be without when venturing into the woods. In Appendix C (page 160) is a checklist for shorter dayhikes and another for longer overnight trips. The lists are intended as a general guide; they include basic gear and some optional items, but are not exhaustive.

If you are new to hiking, spend some time researching appropriate gear that will ensure safe and comfortable hiking in various seasons and trail conditions. Purchase your gear (rental gear is sometimes available) from a reputable outdoor store that specializes in hiking and backpacking; don't attempt to cut corners by visiting a hunting and fishing store and purchasing heavier, often inadequate, equipment made for car camping. Good gear can make the difference between an enjoyable experience and a miserable—or even dangerous—ordeal.

Clothing

Always be prepared for the worst: Bring enough proper clothing to protect you from the most severe weather that is *possible*. Fast-moving cold fronts have been known to drop temperatures in East Texas more than 40 degrees within a few hours. Combine that scenario with heavy rains and high winds, and it is easy to imagine deadly hypothermia, a dangerous drop in body temperature, setting in. It doesn't take freezing temperatures to cause hypothermia.

"Cotton kills" is a common saying in cold climates, but it is just as applicable to hiking in East Texas. Walking in wet cotton clothes on a 45-degree day can easily bring on hypothermia. The key to enjoyable hiking on the LSHT is to layer synthetic clothing. A synthetic shirt, sweater or fleece jacket, and outer shell will keep you both warmer and drier than a single heavy overcoat. Shedding or adding layers enables regulation of body temperature more effectively than a single heavy jacket. Synthetic fabrics dry quickly and maintain their insulating properties when wet. Even in the heat of the summer, it is advisable to wear lightweight synthetic clothing that will dry in the humid conditions of the LSHT. Lightweight long pants and a long-sleeve shirt will protect you from the sun, biting insects, and thorny brush that can overhang the trail.

Footwear

Many a hiking trip has been aborted because of blisters. Footwear is a personal choice that may take some experimenting to master. I prefer to wear midweight leather hiking boots, as well as knee-high synthetic gaiters to keep the mud off of my pant legs, to keep dirt out of my boots, and to protect my lower legs from sharp brush and snakes. Many hikers prefer low-top trail hikers that resemble running shoes. Low-cut gaiters are also available. Whatever your choice of footwear, remember to break in your shoes before you get on the trail. Be comfortable walking through

The Lone Star Hiking Trail

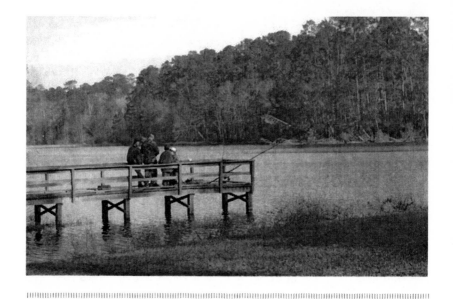

Fishermen at spring-fed Double Lake

shallow water and slippery mud. Don't neglect to purchase high-quality socks made expressly for hiking. On a multiday outing, carry two or three pairs of wool-synthetic blend socks. Consider purchasing quality insoles that provide more support than the standard insoles that come with most shoes.

Sleeping Bags and Pads

A bag rated to 30 or 40°F will probably be adequate for most hikers in the fall and spring. I prefer to carry a warmer sleeping bag (one rated to 20°F) most of the year because I sleep cold. Midsummer on the LSHT can bring extremely hot daytime temperatures, but most people will need at least a light fleece blanket for camping, even in July and August. Summer sleeping bags are lightweight and low cost. Don't forget to bring a sleeping pad, which makes all the difference in warmth and comfort. Pads come in a variety of styles and materials, from cheaper closed cell foam to the more costly inflatable versions. I've used them all, and I do not personally notice a big difference in comfort among the styles available.

Tents

Because of the vigorous insect population in East Texas, I advise using an enclosed tent versus the more open design of a tarp. I have used tarps extensively—and have even slept out in the open under the stars—in drier desert climates, with good results. I tried using a tarp on the LSHT in January, and even though I didn't see any insects during the day and experienced cold temperatures at night, I had to share my sleeping space with a parade of spiders and ants. In warmer seasons, mosquitoes and ticks make an enclosed tent a necessity for comfort.

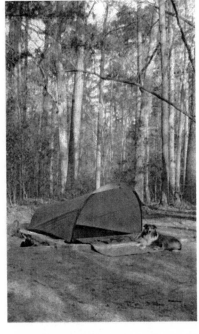

The author's lightweight backpacking tent is home on the trail.

Water Treatment

All water sources harbor microorganisms capable of making you very ill. Carry purification tablets made of iodine or a chlorine compound (the cheapest option) or use a water filter made for hikers. With proper water treatment, you can safely drink just about any water along the LSHT. Obviously, you'll want to avoid filtering or treating very stagnant water or any water draining out of fields that may be contaminated by livestock or pesticides.

Food

Novice hikers often make the mistake of carrying too much food. If you are not accustomed to the exertion of backpacking, your appetite may actually decrease for the first day or two. On the other hand, it is advisable to carry a day of extra food in case you are stranded by bad weather or other trouble. Two pounds of food per person per day is the average. Many lightweight backpacking staples can be purchased at a grocery store; you need not rely on expensive prepared "backpacking food" sold at outdoor stores. See Appendix C (page 160) for specific backpacking food ideas.

Hazards and Personal Safety

Like many outdoor activities, hiking inherently involves some risk. The following is a brief introduction to the most common safety concerns for LSHT hikers. For more instruction on how to administer basic first aid for injuries and illnesses associated with camping, hiking, and backpacking, explore classes and books dedicated to wilderness first aid.

Heat

Heat exhaustion and heat stroke are deadly threats on the LSHT in summer. Carry plenty of water at all times. Take frequent rest breaks when high humidity combines with heat to make it hard for the body to stay cool. Consider hiking only in the lower temperatures of early morning and late evening.

Insects

Bugs may not seem like a real threat, but LSHT hikers are more likely to have an uncomfortable encounter with these creatures than with any other. Both ticks and mosquitoes can carry a variety of life-threatening and debilitating diseases and are present during every month of the year in the moist forests of East Texas.

The worst months for bugs are from April through September. During these warmer months, carry insect repellent and consider wearing long pants. After the first freezing night of the year, usually some time in October, ticks and mosquitoes mostly disappear until the next spring. However, they are present and active year-round. It is a good idea to check for ticks each evening. Removing ticks before they have a chance to feed is important, as several diseases are transmitted only after the tick has been attached at least 24 hours. The diseases that can be transmitted to humans by infected ticks in Texas are: Lyme disease, Rocky Mountain spotted fever, ehrlichiosis, and relapsing fever. If caught early, these diseases can be successfully treated. However, if left untreated, they can be serious or even fatal. Early symptoms may include a rash around the bite or flulike symptoms, such as fever, headache, fatigue, muscle aches, and joint pain.

Chiggers are tiny mites, nearly invisible to humans, which can cause a lot of torment. Most numerous in the spring, chiggers bite into the skin (often around the folds of the body, like the knees or waistline) and cause hard, red welts that itch intensely for up to a week. Your best bet to avoid chiggers is to not sit directly on the ground in the spring and early summer, especially in sunny, grassy areas. Use your tent's ground cloth—or bring along a piece of light plastic—to spread on the ground before you sit down for a break.

Two venomous spider species are found in East Texas: the black widow and the brown recluse. Both species are solitary and live in sheltered areas, such as underneath logs or in thick bushes. Be particularly cautious while off-trail for bathroom activities or collecting firewood—watch where you put your hands. The spiders that build their webs directly across the trail can bite but are not venomous.

Other bothersome insects that hikers may encounter on the LSHT are flies and gnats, especially in mid- to late summer. Fire ants are also present, but typically live in open areas. Watch for their mounds in power line right-of-ways and fields. Of course, bees and wasps are active in all of the warmer months and a serious concern for anyone allergic to their stings.

Snakes

For some hikers, snakes are a major worry. The fact is that snakes offer no real threat to humans—lightning strikes, drowning, and hunting accidents are much more common outdoor hazards. Snakes are an extremely important part of a healthy ecosystem, keeping the population of rodents and small animals in balance. Of the more than 30 species of snakes in East Texas, only a few are venomous: the water moccasin, rattlesnake, copperhead, and coral snake. Look before you sit on logs or against the base of trees. Never reach blindly under logs or into brush. Most snake bites occur on the hands or feet.

Spotting a snake in its natural environment should be treated just like any other wildlife encounter. Keep your distance. Do not kill or try to capture snakes—it is harmful to the environment and potentially harmful to you! Most of those who suffer snakebites are people who handle or approach snakes. Another consideration: Federal and state laws protect a few species of East Texas snakes that are listed as threatened, subjecting violators to fines up to $100,000 or one year of imprisonment.

If the worst happens and you think you've been bitten by a venomous snake, it is important to reach help with a minimum of exertion. Use your maps to find the nearest exit to civilization. Walk out calmly; don't run. Avoid moving the bitten limb more than necessary, and remove any rings or constrictive jewelry before swelling begins. On average, less than 1% of all snake bites recorded in the U.S. are fatal.

Animals

In East Texas bears, jaguars, cougars, and wolves were hunted to extinction by 1950. Coyotes and bobcats are the most numerous large predators in the East Texas woods today; both are extremely timid and will not bother humans. Raccoons are probably the animal most likely to invade hikers' camps in their nightly hunt for food. Hang food in trees away from tree trunks to keep it out of their reach. Most mammals, from coyotes and foxes to skunks and bats, can carry rabies. Do not approach or handle *any* wild animals—for their safety and for yours.

The American alligator has returned in healthy numbers to its home range on the waterways of East Texas. Although they appear frightening, alligators are known to be shy around humans. LSHT hikers have little to fear from them. The best places to watch for the seldom-seen alligators are around the shoreline of Lake Conroe, near Stubblefield, and in the larger waterways, like the San Jacinto River.

Humans

It's a statistical fact that the most dangerous animal encounter a hiker can have is with another human. Hunting accidents happen every year. Even though it is illegal to discharge a weapon across or down a trail corridor, road, or campground, you cannot rule out the possibility that a hunter may fire in your direction or may mistake you for an animal. Wear brightly colored clothing during deer rifle hunting season (November through January) to increase your visibility to hunters.

While you are hiking, keep a low profile. Don't make yourself an easy target for harassment, even though the odds of a person bothering you on the LSHT are extremely low. It's always a good practice not to camp near roads—unless you are in a developed campground—and to camp out of sight of the trail. The idea is not to be paranoid, but to be smart. Watch for traffic while crossing or walking on roads.

Plants

Keep an eye out for poison ivy and poison oak; both are prolific along the LSHT and cause contact dermatitis in most people. Poison ivy is a climbing vine of three leaflets that grows almost straight up instead of twining around its support. Eastern poison oak does indeed have multilobed leaves that resemble oak and can be found in moist, sandy soils. Poison sumac, although not common along the LSHT, is a water-loving tree commonly found in swamps; it is between 6 and 20 feet tall with compound leaves that turn bright red and yellow in the fall. Consult photos of each of these plants before you venture into the East Texas woodland so you can identify them. The branches of these plants (usually bare in winter) can also be poisonous.

From left: poison oak, poison sumac, poison ivy

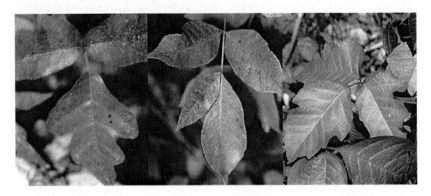

Falling Trees and Limbs

The LSHT's woods are so thick that a hiker may find nowhere to escape falling limbs and trees during high winds. Pine trees have particularly soft wood that splinters easily. Some areas along the trail may even have warnings posted at trailheads informing hikers where there are many standing dead or diseased trees. Always check overhead before pitching a tent in the woods. Look for dead limbs or trees (called "widow-makers") that could fall during the night. Don't venture into the woods during windstorms or when high winds

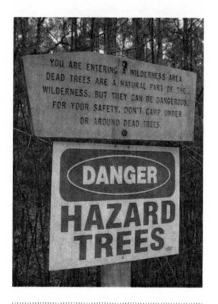

A warning sign posted in the Wilderness Section

are forecast. If you find yourself in the woods during windy conditions, take refuge in a gully or beside large fallen tree trunks that can offer some protection.

Rising Creeks

Heavy rains can cause large creeks and rivers to rise rapidly out of their banks. Dry creek beds and drainages that were once dry may fill up. Bottomlands can turn into extensive swamps. If in doubt about crossing any high water, turn around, or be patient and stay put on dry ground until the water recedes (it may take more than a day or two). During extended periods of rain in late winter, it may be necessary for hikers to detour around flooded areas. However, many sections of the LSHT are located on higher, upland areas away from bottomlands and can be hiked even in very wet weather. Consult the section information in Chapter 3 to identify potential problem areas.

Getting Lost . . . or Misplaced

If you have been walking down the trail and realize that you have not seen any trail markers after about five minutes of hiking, you may want to turn around and retrace your steps until you find a marker. You may have missed a turn in the trail. It's possible that a few trail markers are missing in a section due to vandalism or fallen trees, but the LSHT hiker should never walk more than 5 or 10 minutes without seeing a marker. (A hiker can estimate covering 1 mile in about 30 minutes.) Most of the LSHT road walks are not regularly marked, though, so don't expect to see LSHT trail markers while on roads. Instead, watch your maps and use this book to find your way on road walks.

The forests along the LSHT are often thick and sometimes look the same in every direction, so it is imperative not to wander off the trail into the woods where it's easy to become disoriented. In the event that you do become lost, you have several important decisions to make and some basic guidelines to follow.

First, maintain a calm state of mind. Consider yourself "misplaced" for a bit, not lost. Take a break to think about how long you've been misplaced, what direction you've come from, and what information your map may be able to provide about your location. There are very few places along the LSHT that are more than a long day of walking from a road, a utilities right-of-way, or some form of civilization. Keep your backpack and gear with you at all times. If you are on a trail, don't leave it. It will lead you somewhere much faster and with less danger than trying to walk into the woods off-trail. If you are injured, it is getting dark, or you are panicked or exhausted, make camp and stay put, at least for the night. As a last resort, if you do become lost in deep woods off-trail, follow drainages downstream, or follow utilities or pipeline right-of-ways—eventually, they will lead you to a trail or road.

It is in every hiker's best interest to read a few resources that explain what to do in case you get misplaced while out hiking. Always carry maps and a compass and tell someone back in civilization where you are hiking and when you expect to return home.

chapter three

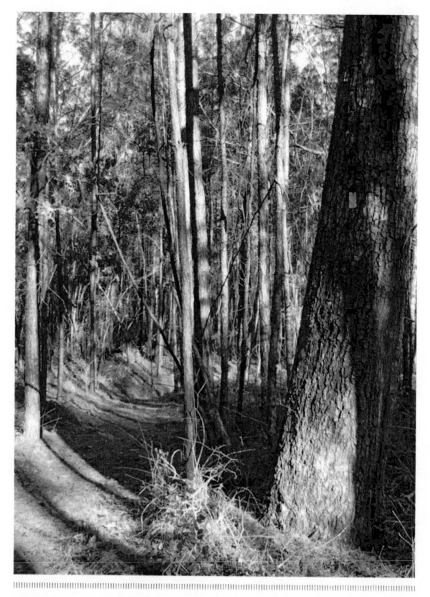

LSHT trail marker on a large oak near the western terminus

trail
sections

**Farm to Market 149 near Richards to
Farm to Market 149 Crossing**

OVERVIEW

The Wilderness Section of the Lone Star Hiking Trail
(LSHT) is so named because it passes through the only
officially designated wilderness area on the trail, 3,855-
acre Little Lake Creek Wilderness, established in 1984.
Protected hardwood bottomland drainages, like Little
Lake Creek, are becoming rare because of pressure
from development, agriculture, logging, and reservoir-
building. Little Lake Creek and its seasonally-flowing
tributaries harbor fertile soils, wetlands, and unique
tree species—an important sanctuary for resident wildlife and migrating waterfowl.

    Hikers in the Wilderness Section experience up-
land pine forests, meandering creeks, palmetto flats,
and seasonal swamps. Water is plentiful, but extensive
boardwalks keep feet dry in most wet areas. Section 1
is both well maintained and easily accessible. A variety
of hiking trails in the area can be linked to make loop
hikes along the LSHT; hikers must pay close attention
to maps and trail markers to avoid losing their way.
A detailed *Little Lake Creek Wilderness* map can be ordered from the U.S. Forest Service; the Sam Houston
National Forest District Office can also provide more
information on other trails in the area (see Appendix
A, page 157).

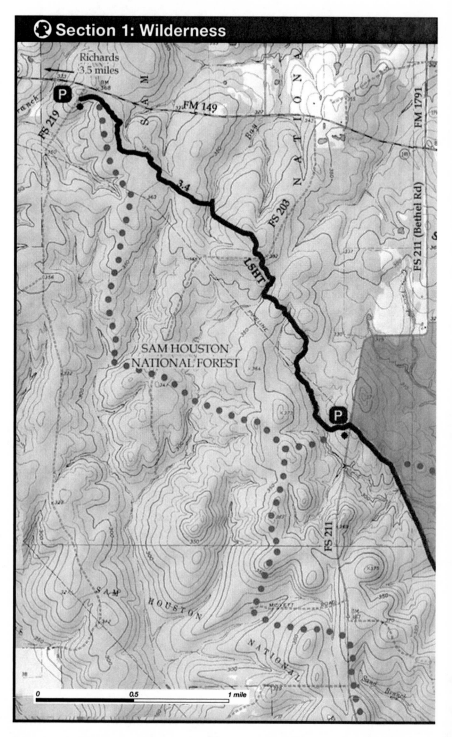

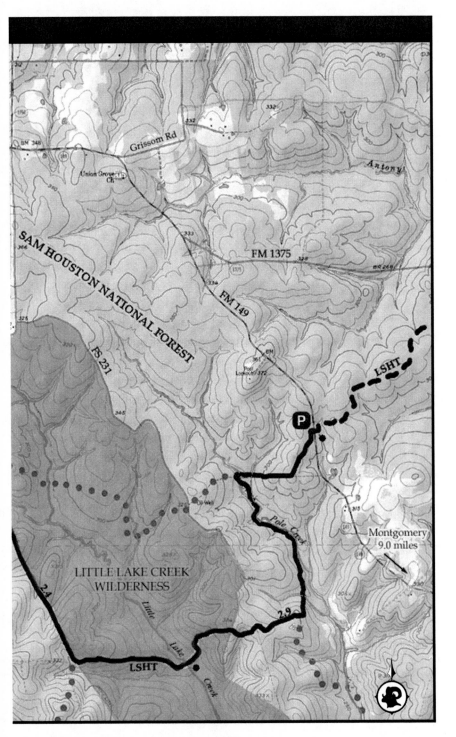

TRAIL ACCESS AND PARKING

Section 1 offers hikers three trailheads with plenty of room for parking. All three areas are located on or near Farm to Market (FM) 149 (designated on signs as Farm Road 149) and have a large gravel parking lot, trash can, and bulletin board posted with trail information. Drinking water is not available at the trailheads.

The western terminus of the LSHT is at the Richards Trailhead Parking Lot #1, approximately 3 miles east of the small town of Richards and 14.5 miles north of Montgomery. Look for the dirt Forest Service (FS) Road 219 on the south side of FM 149. Trailhead Parking Lot #1 is located on the left just 0.1 mile down FS 219. A brown sign on the highway indicates the turnoff for the LONE STAR HIKING TRAIL, but the parking lot is not visible from FM 149.

LSHT Trailhead Parking Lot #2, called Sandy Branch, offers access at trail mile 3.4. Roughly midway between Trailhead Parking Lots #1 and #3 along FM 149, turn onto FS 211 (also called Bethel Road) on the south side of FM 149 (there is no sign for the LSHT at this turn). Trailhead Parking Lot #2 is located on the west side of FS 211 approximately 2 miles from FM 149.

A third trailhead, North Wilderness Trailhead Parking Lot #3, is located on FM 149 about 9.5 miles north of Montgomery where the LSHT crosses FM 149 at trail mile 8.7 at the end of LSHT Section 1. This parking area is signed and visible from the highway.

A potential source of confusion is a fourth trailhead that is signed LONE STAR HIKING TRAIL, but actually connects to the LSHT via the Little Lake Creek Loop Trail. This fourth trailhead, 6.9 miles north of Montgomery, is the first one you see as you drive north on FM 149 from Montgomery.

SECTION 1 GPS Waypoints	
LSHT Richards Trailhead Parking Lot #1 on FM 149	N 30°32.317' W 95°47.090'
LSHT Sandy Branch Trailhead Parking Lot #2 on FS 211	N 30°30.637' W 95°45.420'
Crossing of Little Lake Creek at LSHT Mile 5.9	N 30°29.405' W 95°43.851'
LSHT North Wilderness Trailhead Parking Lot #3 on FM 149	N 30°30.610' W 95°43.079'
Trailhead Parking Lot at Little Lake Creek Loop Trail on FM 149 (not on main LSHT)	N 30°28.912' W 95°41.840'

SUPPLIES AND ACCOMMODATIONS

Richards (population: 300) is 3 miles west of LSHT Trailhead Parking Lot #1, the trail's western terminus, on FM 149. Richards' amenities are limited to two large combination gas station and convenience stores, one of which is named "City Hall" and offers a small cafe. Historic Montgomery (population: 489) is located 9.4 miles south of LSHT Trailhead Parking Lot #3 at trail mile 8.7 at the eastern end of Section 1—at the junction of FM 149 and Texas State Highway (TX) 105. Growing rapidly, it offers more resupply options for hikers, including a full-size grocery store, several restaurants and fast food establishments, gas stations, and many other businesses. At least one bed-and-breakfast offers overnight lodging in Montgomery. Conroe (population: 43,000), 15 miles east of Montgomery on TX 105 along Interstate 45, offers a variety of overnight lodging and services.

WATER

Section 1 frequently follows creeks and passes a small forest pond at mile 2.5. Little Lake Creek flows year-round through seasonal wetlands near mile 6. You can expect to find water at intervals along the way, even in extreme droughts.

TRAIL DESCRIPTION

The LSHT begins in the Sam Houston National Forest beneath a canopy of tall loblolly pines. At **MILE MARKER 1,** open areas in a mature forest of oaks and pines, interspersed with rough jeep tracks, offer possible waterless camping. ▲ As you pass these open sites, the forest undergrowth becomes thicker, limiting camping opportunities until the first creek drainage. Here you will enter into pure stands of immature pines interspersed with recent clear-cuts. You may see evidence of prescribed burns.

Campsite ▲

Around **MILE MARKER 2** there are small seasonal creeks that you first cross, then follow, in a more scenic forest. Clear-cuts and prescribed burns are replaced by wilder, more natural forests. Be careful at mile 2.1 to follow the blazes to the left (remember that if you are westbound, you need to reverse all directions, left and right, in these trail descriptions) heading east-southeast paralleling the dirt road, FS 203, but not crossing it (there may be some conflicting blazes leading northward to the road). Pass an open grassy area beneath smaller trees, top out on a rise under towering pines, and pass a small pond with overgrown banks that offers minimal space for camping. ▲

Campsite ▲

After the pond, the trail parallels a couple of creek drainages and passes some bull pines. The drainage becomes deeper and more apt to hold water as you follow it past **MILE MARKER 3.** There is some relief to the land in the form of several small rises. At mile 3.4, cross over gravel road FS 211 where LSHT Trailhead Parking Lot #2 is visible to the right. Sign the hiker register at the road before entering Little Lake Creek Wilderness. At mile 3.5, past a dense stand of baby pines, there is a clearing off to the right that offers potential camping ▲ out of sight of the road. A boardwalk leads over a wetland, but just a short distance later, a section of unbridged trail near mile 3.7 can be muddy.

▲ **Campsite**

Just before **MILE MARKER 4**, ignore a small section of LSHT that splits into two paths (either way leads quickly to the same outcome), and cross a creek that flows with clear water in the cooler seasons. At mile 4.7, an open area to the right amid well-spaced pines with little understory could make an acceptable dry camp. ▲ A mile later you leave the hardwoods, enter open bottomland where you spot your first dwarf palmettos, and then climb into a pleasant pine upland among giant pines. The rolling landscape drops again into swampy palmetto bottomlands just before **MILE MARKER 5.** Over the course of the next mile, you will be happy to walk on a series of boardwalks built by Boy Scouts. The scenic bottomlands surrounding Little Lake Creek can become a large swamp at times, hiding the creek's exact whereabouts. A new primitive campsite ▲ is reportedly located at mile 5.1, about 0.16 mile off the trail and indicated by aluminum markers painted with a blue tent symbol (there is also a pond in the area that can serve as a water source).

▲ **Campsite**

▲ **Campsite**

Not too far past past **MILE MARKER 6,** ignore an old, abandoned section of trail where a rotting sign lures hikers away from the more modern trail markers. A relatively flat open spot presents itself on the right at mile 6.6, but the trail soon grows brushy as it ascends to a high spot in a tall pine forest. As you near **MILE MARKER 7,** you pass a farm and begin walking downhill along an old barbed wire fence line. Watch for the sharp left turn—be careful not to stay on the ATV track along the fence line. Around the private property expect to hear dogs barking; don't plan to camp in the vicinity.

Campsite ▲

Campsite ▲

You return to a peaceful hardwood forest broken by numerous creeks, one of which the trail follows. There are a few places to scramble down the banks to access water at mile 7.4. Potential campsites ▲ border the creek, although undergrowth becomes thicker at mile 7.5. Native dwarf palmettos and hanging vines lend a junglelike feel to these woods. Just past the bridge at **MILE MARKER 8,** make a right turn to stay on the LSHT at the junction with the North Wilderness Trail, which heads to the left. A camp could be made close to the trail here. ▲ As you gradually climb out of the creek bottom, look for river birch and white oaks before returning to mature upland pine forest. You may hear traffic on FM 149 nearly a mile before you reach the trailhead and LSHT Trailhead Parking Lot #3. Section 2 of the LSHT continues across the highway.

SECTION 1 MILEAGE

MILES W→E	TRAIL POINT	MILES E→W	NOTES
0.0	Western terminus of LSHT; FS 219 at FM 149 LSHT Richards Trailhead Parking Lot #1	96.1	☷ 🅿
0.1	Little Lake Creek Loop Trail (orange-blazed) branches right; follow LSHT left	96.0	
0.2	Utilities right-of-way	95.9	
0.4	Seasonal drainage on left	95.7	
1.0	**MILE MARKER 1**; potential camping	95.1	▲
1.3	Large seasonal drainage	94.8	
1.8	FS 2031A (good dirt road)	94.3	☷
2.0	Small seasonal drainage; **MILE MARKER 2**	94.1	
2.1	LSHT blazed in two directions; follow LSHT left parallel to FS 203 (good dirt road)	94.0	☷
2.2	Abandoned jeep road	93.9	
2.5	Small pond (semi-clear water); potential camping	93.6	🍶 ▲
2.7	ATV/jeep track; large seasonal drainage	93.4	
3.0	**MILE MARKER 3**	93.1	

SECTION 1 MILEAGE

MILES W→E	TRAIL POINT	MILES E→W	NOTES
3.3	Junction with West Fork Trail; large seasonal drainage	92.8	
3.4	FS 211 (good gravel road); LSHT Sandy Branch Trailhead Parking Lot #2; enter Little Lake Creek (LLC) Wilderness	92.7	▬ P
3.5	Potential camping	92.6	▲
3.7	Hiker gate at a fence	92.4	
3.8	Wilderness Trail branches left; follow LSHT straight	92.3	
4.0	MILE MARKER 4; creek (low volume; good water)	92.1	⛲*
4.6	Large seasonal drainage (stagnant water)	91.5	
4.7	Potential camping	91.4	▲
5.0	MILE MARKER 5	91.1	
5.1	Intersect Sand Branch Trail; follow LSHT left; LLC Wilderness boundary	91.0	
5.8	Old (inaccurate) wooden milepost "6"	90.3	
5.9	Boardwalks over Little Lake Creek bottomland	90.2	
6.0	MILE MARKER 6	90.1	
6.5	LLC Wilderness boundary; jeep road	89.6	
6.7	ATV track on right	89.4	
6.8	Pole Creek Trail (blue-blazed) to right; follow LSHT left	89.3	
7.0	MILE MARKER 7	89.1	
7.2	Creek adjacent to trail (low volume; good water)	88.9	⛲*
7.7	Hiker bridge over deep drainage	88.4	
7.9	Old wooden milepost "8"	88.2	
8.0	MILE MARKER 8; potential camping; creek (low volume; good water)	88.1	⛲ ▲
8.6	Utilities right-of-way	87.5	
8.7	FM 149 LSHT North Wilderness Trailhead Parking Lot #3	87.4	▬ P

Water here is seasonal and dependent on weather conditions.

MILEAGE CHART KEY

⛲	Water source	▲	Undeveloped campsite or potential camping area
🚐	Developed campground		
P	Parking area/trailhead	▬▬	Major roads (jeep tracks and logging roads are not indicated)

Farm to Market 149 Crossing to
Farm to Market 1375

OVERVIEW

Hikers in the Kelly Section will enjoy walking through a wide variety of forest communities. The Caney Creek bottomlands, in particular, offer an enjoyable mix of tree species and plant communities that harbor an abundance of birds and wildlife. This section offers few reliable water sources for overnight hikers, but tends to remain muddy in many areas. All large creeks are bridged and the trail continues to be easy to follow, with abundant trail markers and signs. There are plenty of high and dry campsites to be found along the way, though hikers may need to carry water to camp.

The intersection of the Lone Star Hiking Trail (LSHT) and Little Lake Creek Loop Trail offers hikers a chance to walk a large loop that connects Sections 1 and 2. A detailed *Little Lake Creek Wilderness* map can be ordered from the U.S. Forest Service; the Sam Houston National Forest District Office can also provide more information (see Appendix A, page 157) about this loop hike.

TRAIL ACCESS AND PARKING

Section 2 offers hikers two official LSHT trailhead parking areas with large gravel parking lots, trash cans, and bulletin boards posted with trail information. Additionally, there is trailside parking at the LSHT crossing of Osborn Road (Forest Service Road 237) at mile 11.3 and Forest Service Road 271 (just off of Forest Service Road 204) at mile 14.4. Potable water is not available at the trailheads.

The western end of Section 2 at mile 8.7 offers parking in the LSHT North Wilderness Trailhead Parking Lot #3 on Farm to Market (FM) 149 (designated on signs as Farm Road 149) about 9.5 miles north of Montgomery where the LSHT crosses FM 149. The eastern end of Section 2 offers hiker parking at the LSHT Stubblefield Trailhead Parking Lot #6 just off of Farm to Market 1375 down a small dirt access road (the parking lot is not visible from the highway) at LSHT mile 15.8. Both parking areas/trail crossings are well-signed.

SECTION 2 GPS Waypoints	
LSHT North Wilderness Trailhead Parking Lot #3 on FM 149	N 30°30.610' W 95°43.079'
LSHT Trailhead Parking Lot on Little Lake Creek Loop	N 30°28.912' W 95°41.840'
Crossing of Caney Creek at mile 11.9	N 30°31.241' W 95°40.619'
LSHT Stubblefield Trailhead Parking Lot #6 on FM 1375	N 30°31.563' W 95°37.812'

SUPPLIES AND ACCOMMODATIONS

Montgomery (population: 489) is 9.4 miles south of the North Wilderness Trailhead Parking Lot #3 on FM 149 at the beginning of Section 2. Montgomery is a full-service town that offers a grocery store, several restaurants, gas stations, and many other businesses. At least one bed-and-breakfast offers overnight lodging in Montgomery. Conroe (population: 43,000), 15 miles east of Montgomery on Texas State Highway (TX) 105 along Interstate 45, offers a wide variety of overnight lodging and services.

At the end of Section 2, New Waverly (population: 950) lies approximately 9 miles east of the Stubblefield Parking Lot #6 on FM 1375 (just east of I-45). New Waverly does not offer any overnight lodging, but does host several combination gas station and convenience stores, restaurants, an auto parts store, a library,

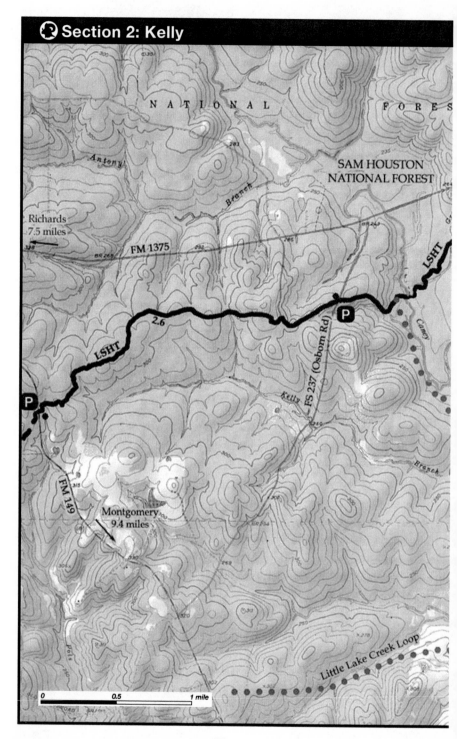

NATIONAL   FORES

SAM HOUSTON
NATIONAL FOREST

Richards
7.5 miles

FM 1375

Branch

LSHT

2.6

LSHT

FS 237 (Osborn Rd.)

Kelly

P

Caney

Branch

FM 149

Montgomery
9.4 miles

Little Lake Creek Loop

0   0.5   1 mile

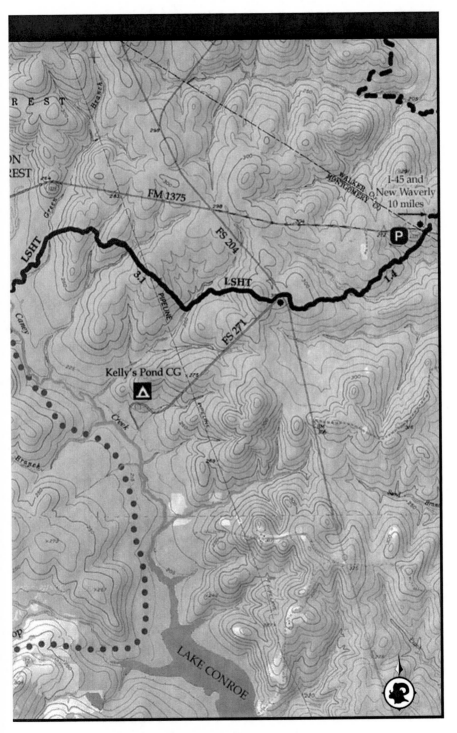

and a grocery store. From New Waverly, it is 15 miles north on I-45 to the full-service town of Huntsville, which offers many options for overnight lodging.

WATER

Water is not as regular in Section 2 as it is in Section 1. Plan your hike carefully if you need water for camping. Although there are plenty of campsites, most of them are in dry areas. The most reliable water source in this section is Caney Creek at mile 11.9. In fact, in dry times, this may be the only water on the LSHT in the Kelly Section.

TRAIL DESCRIPTION

Section 2 begins at LSHT Trailhead Parking Lot #3 on FM 149 at mile 8.7. From this dirt parking lot, as you are standing near the information board, look directly across FM 149. You should be able to see the trail

A hiker next to a huge pine tree in the Kelly Section

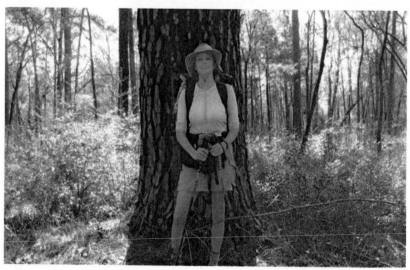

marked on the other side of the highway where it heads into the woods. After crossing FM 149, the trail swings to the left along an old barbed wire fence, crosses a jeep track and makes a hard right turn. (Remember that if you are westbound, you need to reverse all directions, left and right, in these trail descriptions.) At mile 8.9, you reach a junction of trails where the blazes may be hard for eastbound trekkers to see. The LSHT makes a sharp left turn here. Shortly, after the turn, **MILE MARKER 9** is visible on a tree to the right of the trail. Again, at mile 9.1, the LSHT makes another hard turn—this one to the left—as it reaches a faint jeep track that continues straight. It would be easy to miss this turn, so watch carefully.

Yet another junction of trails at mile 9.3 is clearly marked; the LSHT heads off to the left and soon reaches some flat land in an open forest that could be used for waterless camping. ▲ At mile 9.6 the trail begins   **▲ Campsite** to skirt a young pine forest to the right but stays within the canopy of the larger oak–pine forest to the left. If it has been raining a lot, there may be some standing water in this area. As you begin to cross a maze of normally dry gullies at mile 9.8, a small pond may be visible on the left just before you reach an undefined path that crosses the LSHT at a large downed log, making a nice break spot.

As you pass **MILE MARKER 10,** keep an eye out for one of the first giant oaks adjacent to the LSHT. An enormous pine on the right also begs attention at mile 10.3. Around mile 10.5 there may be a few open spaces to the right for a waterless campsite. ▲ One of the old,   **▲ Campsite** outdated wooden posts inscribed with a barely perceptible 11 is actually located at mile 10.8. Soon after, at mile 10.9, pass an old fence with an out-of-use hiker gate and make a right turn at a T-junction of trails just before **MILE MARKER 11**. An old roadbed makes for good tread in a mature pine forest until you reach Osborn Road at mile 11.3.

Osborn Road (Forest Service Road 237) is an unstriped paved road that offers a few parking spots. The LSHT is well marked at this road junction. FM 1375 is located to the left (north) less than a mile up Osborn Road. In the springtime, the air here is full of the scent of honeysuckle as you head back into the woods and cross a utilities right-of-way, passing beneath overhead wires. Do you remember intersecting the Little Lake Creek Loop Trail just after you began hiking at the western terminus of the LSHT? Now you have reached its other end, at mile 11.8, where it is well signed and blazed with orange markers. The LSHT continues straight ahead, while the Little Lake Creek Loop heads off to the right and back toward the LSHT's western terminus.

The author's dog, Buddy, cools off in the clear waters of Caney Creek beneath the LSHT footbridge.

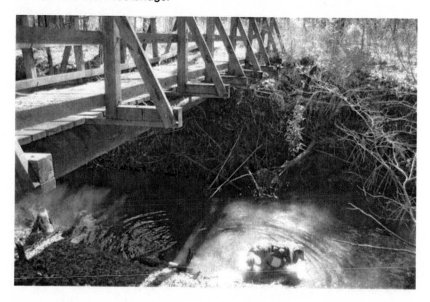

Immediately, you head down to Caney Creek, normally flowing with clear water on its way to Lake Conroe only 2 miles downstream. Quiet hikers may walk up on wood ducks enjoying the clean creek water. In this hardwood bottomland grows a variety of vegetation: dwarf palmettos, oaks, and hanging vines. A lone mature pine rises a hundred feet above scattered river cane, one of three temperate bamboo species native to North America. These flat seasonal bottomlands can also be covered with thick grasses that obscure the LSHT. Luckily, trail markers are plentiful in this area. This low area is usually muddy, but in dry times there are several potential campsites ▲ along the creek.

▲ **Campsite**

MILE MARKER 12 is in a picturesque grove of large oaks hung with Spanish moss, which is not actually a true moss but a bromeliad and relative of the pineapple! This moss does not typically harm its host trees and provides a home to insects, snakes, and some species of bats. In the past, Native Americans used Spanish moss for clothing and medicinal purposes, while pioneers used it to caulk cabins and stuff saddle blankets. At mile 12.2, you cross a dry drainage that has the potential to hold quite a bit of runoff during wet weather. Look for more palmettos, river cane, and the shortest-lived oak species, the water oak (*Quercus nigra*). With a lifespan of 60 to 80 years, the large water oaks seen here are nearing old age.

Near mile 12.5, the trail rises up out of the swampy bottomland onto a pine-dominated upland. The path continues to climb until it crosses a heavily used ATV track at the top of a hill. A small creek that usually has flowing clear water is crossed soon afterward. The old wooden milepost 13 is actually fairly near to the contemporary **MILE MARKER 13.** You cross another creek—this one usually dry—on a small,

leaning bridge, and then top a gentle rise in an open forest of mature pines. Hikers could make camp just
Campsite ▲ about anywhere in this mature pine plantation, ▲ although there is no water nearby.

A good gravel road suitable for high-clearance vehicles crosses the trail parallel to a pipeline right-of-way at mile 13.3. Expect the bridged creek at mile 13.7 to be dry most of the time. The trail becomes a bit muddy and increasingly brushy and difficult to see as you pass MILE MARKER 14. However, frequent trail markers make navigating easy in this often overgrown area; just keep looking for them on the trees ahead as you hike. At mile 14.2, cross a well-used ATV track and ascend to a unique, picturesque hilltop view at mile 14.3, from which you can see a dirt road ahead and below. At the dirt road, FS 271, there is a bit of impromptu parking and a garbage can; eastbound hikers should watch for a diagonal blaze leading them back into the woods on the LSHT.

One mile to the right on FS 271 is Kelly's Pond
Campsite ▲ Campground. ▲ Popular with hunters, this campground offers eight primitive campsites with picnic tables, fire rings, and a pit toilet (no potable water or electricity; possible fee). To the left, the LSHT follows FS 271 a short distance to the unstriped, but paved FS 204. Veer to the right and cross over this paved road, following the LSHT HIKERS ONLY sign back into the woods. At mile 14.5, you cross an abandoned road in mixed woodland. Another sign leads you across a large ATV track at mile 14.7. Soon, the trail crosses a smaller bike track as it nears a house. Dogs may begin barking as you hike past the private property, making the wide, flat open areas impractical as campsites. Two more undefined trails intersect the LSHT. The attractive riparian area that follows, with its diversity of hardwood trees, offers a good lunch or break spot.

Just before reaching **MILE MARKER 15,** there are a few open areas peaceful enough to warrant camping. ▲ Sand Creek, usually filled with shallow murky water, is just beyond; the trail follows along its banks and then crosses it at mile 15.1. Large loblolly pines appear as the trail heads into a sloping upland. A small sandy-bottomed creek at mile 15.6 may harbor a trickle of water. You reach FM 1375 at mile 15.8, the end of Section 2. Ahead is a dirt road that leads to LSHT Trailhead Parking Lot #6. The trail continues into the woods just to the right of the dirt road on the other side of FM 1375.

▲ **Campsite**

SECTION 2 MILEAGE

MILES W→E	TRAIL POINT	MILES E→W	NOTES
8.7	FM 149; LSHT North Wilderness Trailhead Parking Lot #3	87.4	☷ 🅿
8.9	Junction of trails; follow LSHT left	87.2	
9.0	**MILE MARKER 9**	87.1	
9.1	Jeep track; follow LSHT left	87.0	
9.3	Junction of trails; follow LSHT left	86.8	
9.8	Pond (hard to see) on left	86.3	
10.0	**MILE MARKER 10**	86.1	
10.5	Potential waterless campsites	85.6	▲
10.9	T-junction; follow LSHT right	85.2	
11.0	**MILE MARKER 11**	85.1	
11.3	Osborn Road (FS 237); trailhead parking	84.8	☷ 🅿
11.4	Utilities right-of-way	84.7	
11.8	Little Lake Creek Loop branches right; follow LSHT straight ahead	84.3	
11.9	Caney Creek (high volume; good water); potential camping	84.2	🚰 ▲
12.0	**MILE MARKER 12;** swampy area	84.1	
12.2	Large seasonal drainage	83.9	
12.7	ATV track at top of hill	83.4	
12.8	Creek (low volume; good water)	83.3	🚰*

SECTION 2 MILEAGE

MILES W→E	TRAIL POINT	MILES E→W	NOTES
13.0	Old wooden milepost; **MILE MARKER 13**	83.1	
13.1	Seasonal creek	83.0	
13.3	Pipeline right-of-way; gravel access road	82.8	
13.7	Creek (stagnant water)	82.4	
14.0	**MILE MARKER 14**	82.1	
14.2	ATV track	81.9	
14.4	FS 271 (good dirt road); FS 204 (paved road); Kelly's Pond Campground 1 mile right on FS 271	81.7	▬ 🚐
14.7	ATV track	81.4	
15.0	**MILE MARKER 15;** potential camping; creek (low volume; murky)	81.1	🚰 ▲
15.6	Seasonal creek	80.5	
15.8	FM 1375; LSHT Stubblefield Trailhead Parking Lot #6	80.3	▬ 🅿

* Water here is seasonal and dependent on weather conditions.

MILEAGE CHART KEY

🚰 Water source

🚐 Developed campground

🅿 Parking area/trailhead

▲ Undeveloped campsite or potential camping area

▬▬ Major roads (jeep tracks and logging roads are not indicated)

Farm to Market 1375 Crossing to Cotton Creek Cemetery Road

OVERVIEW

Highlights of the Conroe Section include a large, view-filled waterfront camping area on the shore of Lake Conroe, as well as the picturesque and peaceful Stubblefield Lake Campground along old Stubblefield Lake. Both areas offer good wildlife viewing and opportunities to fish. The region between these two highlights also takes hikers into swampy areas that, in wet seasons, can mean wading through calf-deep water for short stretches, but also mean experiencing a lush ecosystem different from any other on the LSHT. However, the majority of Section 3 is on high and dry ground, where very few water sources are available. This section ends with a 2-mile road walk that follows peaceful country roads, taking hikers past historic ranches and farms. As noted in the trail description, several areas lack regular trail markers and require careful attention.

TRAIL ACCESS AND PARKING

Only one official parking lot serves Section 3. LSHT Stubblefield Trailhead Parking Lot #6 at LSHT mile 15.8 is located off of Farm to Market (FM) 1375 down a small dirt access road (the parking lot is not visible from the highway, but is well-signed) at LSHT mile 15.8. Potable water is not available here.

In addition, there is a large dirt parking area on Forest Service (FS) Road 215 just across from the trail at LSHT mile 20.3, near the road bridge over Stubblefield Lake (FS 215 can be accessed from FM 1375 a few miles west of LSHT Stubblefield Trailhead Parking Lot

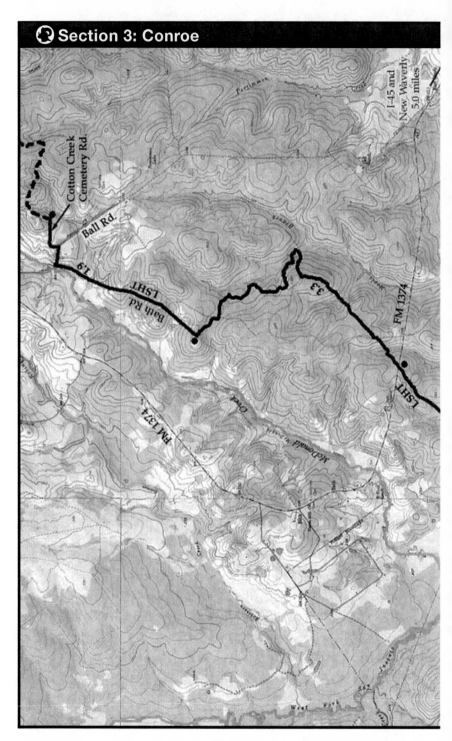

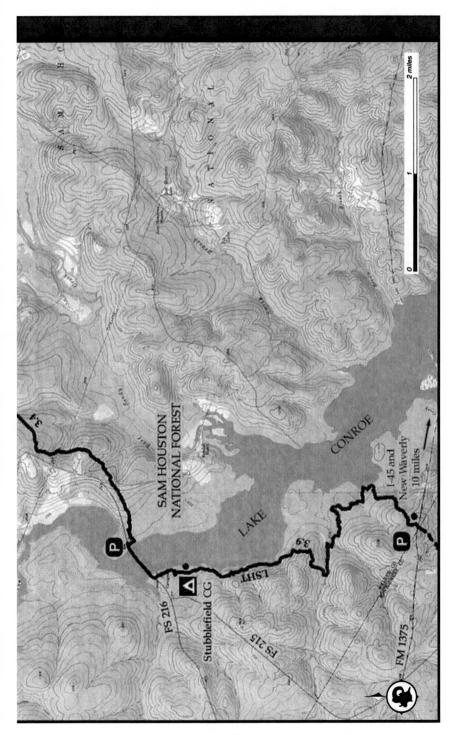

SAM HOUSTON
NATIONAL FOREST

SAM H...

NATIONAL

LAKE

CONROE

I-45 and
New Waverly
10 miles

FS 216

Stubblefield CG

FS 215

LSHT

FM 1375

3.4

3.9

2 miles

1

0

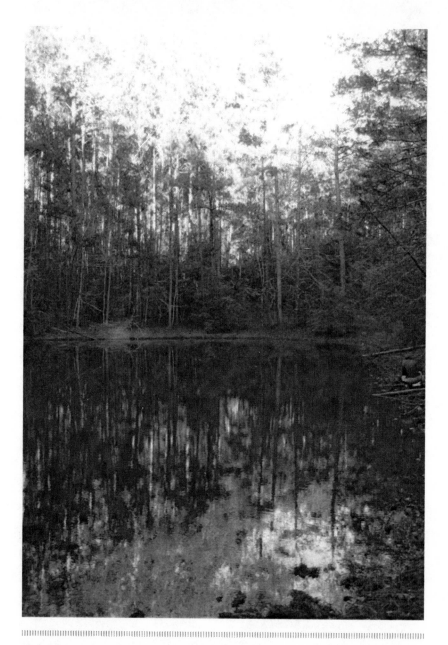

The LSHT passes this small pond at the western end of the Conroe Section.

#6). This unofficial parking lot is adjacent to Stubble-
field Lake Campground, where it is possible to acquire
drinking water. Parking a vehicle in the campground
requires a daily fee of $5.

SECTION 3 GPS Waypoints	
LSHT Stubblefield Trailhead Parking Lot #6 on FM 1375	N 30°31.563' W 95°37.812'
Stubblefield Lake Campground	N 30°33.536' W 95°38.228'
FM 1374 at LSHT mile 23.1	N 30°35.253' W 95°36.293'
Intersection of Bath and Ball Roads	N 30°38.040' W 95°35.378'
Beginning of Cotton Creek Cemetery Road	N 30°38.015' W 95°35.218'

SUPPLIES AND ACCOMMODATIONS

At the west end of Section 3 at LSHT mile 15.8, New
Waverly (population: 950) lies approximately 9 miles
east of the Stubblefield Parking Lot #6 on FM 1375
(just east of Interstate 45). New Waverly does not offer
any overnight lodging, but does offer several combination gas station and convenience stores, restaurants,
an auto parts store, a library, and a grocery store. From
New Waverly, it is 15 miles north on I-45 to the full-
service town of Huntsville, which offers many options
for overnight lodging.

The developed Stubblefield Lake Campground at
LSHT mile 19.7 offers pay phones, restrooms with running water and hot showers, and tent pads (fee of $10 per
campsite). Although a small grocery store used to be located near Stubblefield, it is no longer in business. There
are no vending machines located at this campground.

WATER

Only two reliable sources of water are found in Section
3 directly on the trail: the Lake Conroe shoreline at

mile 16.5 and Stubblefield Lake Campground at mile 19.7. Other creeks and seasonal drainages along the way will contain water in wet seasons, but should not be relied upon during hot or dry months.

TRAIL DESCRIPTION

Section 3 starts at the LSHT crossing of FM 1375. As the trail reenters the woods here, it quickly intersects a well-signed side trail heading off to the left that leads to LSHT Parking Lot #6. You continue on the main path, gradually climbing through a mature pine forest with a thick undergrowth of yaupon and honeysuckle. Just a few minutes past **MILE MARKER 16**, the trail heads downhill, toward 22,000-acre Lake Conroe, which was built in 1972. The lake comes into view at mile 16.5. Along the shoreline, a large open area beneath big pines is a

The view of Lake Conroe through the trees from the large waterfront campsite at mile 16.5

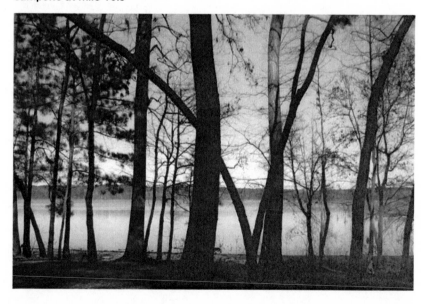

perfect spot for camping, ▲ complete with a nice view **▲ Campsite**
and easy access to the lake. At least, plan to take a break
here; there won't be a better spot until you reach Stubblefield Lake Campground at 19.7. Among the trees on
the shoreline, you may be able to spot the heart-shaped
leaves of the linden (also called the basswood), a large
shade tree native to Asia, Europe, and eastern North
America. You may also want to keep an eye out for bald
eagles, which have been known to nest in this area.

As you leave the shoreline, make a left turn to
follow the LSHT eastbound. (Remember that if you
are westbound, you need to reverse all directions, left
and right, in these trail descriptions.) Cross a gully
and parallel it until you cross it again at mile 16.8.
Although water in this gully is usually not flowing
well, it may offer a more appealing (less silt-laden)
source as opposed to Lake Conroe. Brushy yaupon
thickets mix here with open, palmetto-filled flats. At
MILE MARKER 17, the lake is again visible through the
trees to the right. There are two decent flat sites for
camping ▲ at miles 17.1 and 17.3. A seasonal creek **▲ Campsite**
intersects the LSHT at mile 17.5, which marks entry
into an extensive swampy area. If you find water over
the trail, be patient, expect to get a little wet, and make
your way around and through it as carefully as you
can. The trail soon reaches drier ground again, and
you may see some interesting trees and animal life. In
particular, the endangered red-cockaded woodpecker
may be seen, or heard, in this area.

At mile 17.7 there is an open place across a big
creek that appears to be mowed. The creek stays next to
the LSHT for a bit and contains unusually clear water.
Cross this creek at mile 17.9 on a nice bridge, then cross
a seasonal drainage and pass **MILE MARKER 18**. A wide
jeep trail in decent condition, though not heavily used,

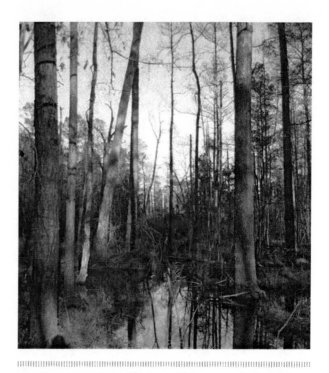

The wetland alongside the trail at mile 17.5

appears at mile 18.3. The well-signed LSHT crosses this track diagonally to the left, and there is an opening adjacent to the road where a waterless camp ▲ could be made (you are not far from the lakeshore in this area and may even spot a few unofficial side trails to the right of the LSHT that lead down to the water). The trail meanders into a jungly area at mile 18.6, but soon reenters a forest of big oaks and pines. Lake Conroe can again be seen off to the right. **MILE MARKER 19** is located just after the trail dips into a grassy, swampy bottomland sporting profuse gardens of dwarf palmettos.

Campsite ▲

The footbridge at mile 19.2 may still be in disrepair; if so, look for downed logs to help make the crossing easier. Giant pine trees draw your attention upward. As you pass by an old clear-cut to the left, a side trail on the right appears to lead down to the lakeshore. The LSHT heads onward over two small hiker bridges that span seasonal creeks in picturesque forests of sweetgum, water oak, hickory, and American holly (*Ilex opaca*), the latter of which reaches its greatest size in these East Texas forests.

At mile 19.7, you leave the woods and enter the developed Stubblefield Lake Campground. ▲ For a fee of $10 per campsite, the campground offers restrooms with running water, hot showers, potable water taps, and clean campsites with picnic tables and tent pads. A pay phone is also located in the campground. Stubblefield Lake is now an arm of Lake Conroe, but it was originally built by the Civilian Conservation Corps (CCC) in 1937 as part of President Franklin D. Roosevelt's New Deal programs.

▲ Campsite

From where the LSHT enters Stubblefield Lake Campground, take a right on the paved campground road and follow it past the picnic pavilion and restroom building. You should see LSHT trail markers leading you in this direction. When you reach the unpaved road (FS 215) and leave the campground behind, take a right and walk over the short road bridge that is usually host to several people fishing for largemouth bass, crappie, bluegill, and catfish. You may also see kayakers and canoeists enjoying this peaceful part of the lake that is too shallow for motorized boats. This is a good spot along the LSHT to look for alligators, wintering bald eagles, and osprey (fishing eagles). Along this road, you pass **MILE MARKER 20**. After crossing the bridge, a large parking area comes into view on the left, and the LSHT reenters the woods at mile 20.3 through a fence line on the right. A few minutes later, make a sharp left turn, avoiding the old trail that continues straight ahead.

Campsite ▲

Just past **MILE MARKER 21** is a small open site followed by an unstriped, paved road and a utilities right-of-way. The trail remains well marked through here. At mile 21.3, cross a seasonal drainage in a pretty area of thick pine, oak, and yaupon. An unmarked trail veers off to the right, and then an ATV track intersects the LSHT. There are some flat spots with room for tents ▲ at mile 21.5, but this area is near a dirt road leading to some trailer homes. Continue onward past a few more dry gullies on brushy trail, past a firebreak or pipeline, and around several more gullies. A larger creek is crossed at mile 21.9 and may offer some clear, flowing water.

MILE MARKER 22 is high in a tree and difficult to spot; once you reach an old deer stand on the left near trees painted with red marks, you have passed the mile marker. Just ahead is an open borderline of property boundaries and some big trees, but this quickly gives way to very thick undergrowth. The LSHT tunnels through the brush while huge pines tower overhead. At mile 22.2 cross a creek that has a stony bottom, something not often seen in East Texas. Pass old milepost 22 and then make a right onto an overgrown jeep track. There are very few trail markers along the old road, but you follow it for a while. Cross another normally dry, rocky-bottomed creek and then reach a split in the road at mile 22.6. The LSHT takes the left fork, and the woods begin to open up more, even offering a few potential waterless campsites. At mile 22.9, reach a barbed wire fence that marks private property (a farmstead) on the left. Try to ignore the trash that seems to accumulate as you pass **MILE MARKER 23**. Very soon you reach the intersection of the LSHT with FM 1374; cross the highway diagonally to the right and reenter the woods at a hiker gate on the other side of the road. There is no trailhead parking along FM 1374.

After crossing a few small seasonal creeks in an open forest, turn left onto a fairly large dirt road. Walking down this road, you should see trail markers that lead you back into the woods on the right side of the road. Reach a larger creek that may harbor water and would make a nice camping spot just before **MILE MARKER 24**. At mile 24.5, take a right onto a seldom-used dirt road. At mile 24.7 a trail marked with two white blazes heads off to the right. Although the markers may appear similar to LSHT markers, stay on the road until you spot the LSHT heading into the woods to the left of the road.

In a young pine forest, pass **MILE MARKER 25**. A large seasonal drainage, an old logging road, and possible dry camping in some open flats are passed in the next half mile. At mile 25.5, an unusually large oak tree catches the eye just before a dry ditch. Keep an eye out for red maple trees in the next mile or so; true to their name, they turn a deep scarlet in fall. The trail tread is not easy to see in this area, but trail markers dutifully lead the way. On the right, several large gullies and creeks come together at mile 25.9. A nice (maybe waterless) camp ▲ could be made here. Just a few minutes after passing **MILE MARKER 26**, turn right onto a jeep track. Trail markers may be a little underused through here; stay on the main track. At mile 26.4, pass through an old broken gate and make a right onto the historic (dirt) Bath Road. As you walk the next 1.5 miles down Bath Road, you'll pass **MILE MARKER 27**, as well as farms (including the Harding Ranch, which claims it was established in 1850), houses, and horse pastures. You will also cross MacDonald Creek, but it is most likely polluted from livestock runoff and is not recommended as a water source.

▲ Campsite

As you reach the intersection of Bath and Ball roads at mile 27.9, make a right onto paved Ball Road. LSHT trail markers lead the way past **MILE MARKER 28**, which may not be visible from the road. As you top a small rise, you come to a white gravel road on the right at mile 28.1; this may appear to be a private drive but it is, in fact, Cotton Creek Cemetery Road, and you will need to turn left onto it. *If you continue on paved Ball Road, which swings to the right here, you may end up walking a long way before you realize your error!* There are only a few trail markers along Cotton Creek Cemetery Road. At mile 28.3, after crossing a second cattle grate, you will see a green house on the right, followed by a newer brick home. It may feel as if you are walking up their driveway, but soon the road swings to the left and deteriorates to an old, little-used jeep track. A sign lets you know that you are entering the national forest again at mile 28.4, officially the end of Section 3 and the beginning of Section 4.

Approaching the junction of Cotton Creek Cemetery and Ball roads in the Conroe Section

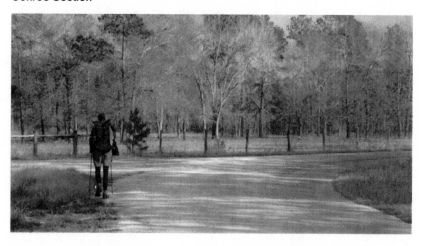

SECTION 3 MILEAGE			
MILES W→E	TRAIL POINT	MILES E→W	NOTES
15.8	FM 1375; LSHT Stubblefield Trailhead Parking Lot #6	80.3	➽ 🅿
16.0	**MILE MARKER 16**	80.1	
16.5	Lake Conroe shoreline; large campsite	79.6	🚰 ⛺
16.8	Creek (medium volume; slow-flowing, semi-clear water)	79.3	🚰
17.0	**MILE MARKER 17**	79.1	
17.3	Potential campsite	78.8	⛺
17.5	Seasonal drainage; wetlands	78.6	
17.9	Large creek (medium volume; good water)	78.2	🚰
18.0	Cross seasonal drainage; **MILE MARKER 18**	78.1	
18.3	Jeep trail; potential campsites	77.8	⛺
19.0	**MILE MARKER 19**	77.1	
19.2	Swampy creek (stagnant water)	76.9	
19.7	Stubblefield Lake Campground	76.4	➽ 🚰 🅿 🚻
20.0	FS 215 road bridge; **MILE MARKER 20**	76.1	➽
20.3	End road walk and reenter woods to right of road	75.8	
21.0	**MILE MARKER 21;** unstriped, paved road; utilities right-of-way	75.1	➽
21.4	ATV track	74.7	
21.5	Potential campsites	74.6	⛺
21.7	Fire break or pipeline right-of-way	74.4	
21.9	Seasonal creek	74.2	
22.0	**MILE MARKER 22;** property boundary; potential campsites	74.1	⛺
22.2	Stony-bottomed seasonal creek; wooden milepost 22	73.9	
22.3	Turn right onto old jeep track	73.8	
22.6	Jeep road splits; take left fork	73.5	
23.0	Private farm on left; **MILE MARKER 23**	73.1	
23.1	FM 1374	73.0	➽
23.5	Turn left onto large dirt road for a few hundred feet	72.6	
24.0	**MILE MARKER 24;** potential campsite	72.1	⛺
24.5	Turn right onto dirt road for 0.2 mile	71.6	
24.7	Turn left onto LSHT and reenter woods	71.4	

SECTION 3 MILEAGE

MILES W→E	TRAIL POINT	MILES E→W	NOTES
25.0	**MILE MARKER 25**	71.1	
25.2	Large seasonal drainage	70.9	
25.3	Old logging road	70.8	
26.0	Potential campsite; **MILE MARKER 26**	70.1	▲
26.1	Take a right onto jeep track	70.0	
26.4	Old metal gate; turn right onto dirt Bath Road	69.7	▬
27.0	**MILE MARKER 27** along Bath Road	69.1	
27.9	Intersection of Bath and Ball Roads; turn right onto Ball Road	68.2	▬
28.0	**MILE MARKER 28** along Ball Road	68.1	
28.1	Turn left onto gravel Cotton Creek Cemetery Road	68.0	▬
28.3	National forest property boundary; swing left on old dirt road	67.7	

MILEAGE CHART KEY

   Water source   ▲ Undeveloped campsite or potential camping area

   Developed campground

   Parking area/trailhead   ▬▬▬ Major roads (jeep tracks and logging roads are not indicated)

Cotton Creek Cemetery Road to Evelyn Lane

OVERVIEW

Although the Huntsville Section of the Lone Star Hiking Trail (LSHT) includes more road walks than any other, one of which has the hiker walking along and beneath Interstate 45, it still has a lot to offer. The walking is pleasant and enjoyable through classic piney woods, but country road walks and the crossing of Camelia Lake provide a break in the monotony of the thick woods. The LSHT follows the large creek named Alligator Branch for more than a mile. A wide variety of water-loving trees, like sycamore, and numerous resident and seasonal bird species can be found in this area.

Hikers should have little trouble following the trail's route in Section 4. Only the trail around the west end of Alligator Branch offers a challenge; even in relatively dry seasons, expect to get your feet muddy for a few minutes while walking through this rich swampland.

The LSHT never enters the boundaries of 2,000-acre Huntsville State Park, but it is near enough to the park to offer LSHT hikers further recreational opportunities. Paddling the park's lake in a rented canoe, or biking and walking its trails, makes an excellent diversion within a few miles of the LSHT. Those who are thru-hiking will want to resupply, or at least grab a hot shower at Huntsville State Park, or along I-45 where there are several reasonably priced motel chains and restaurants about 4.5 miles north of the trailhead.

TRAIL ACCESS AND PARKING

There is no parking area on Cotton Creek Cemetery Road at the west end of Section 4 at LSHT mile 28.3.

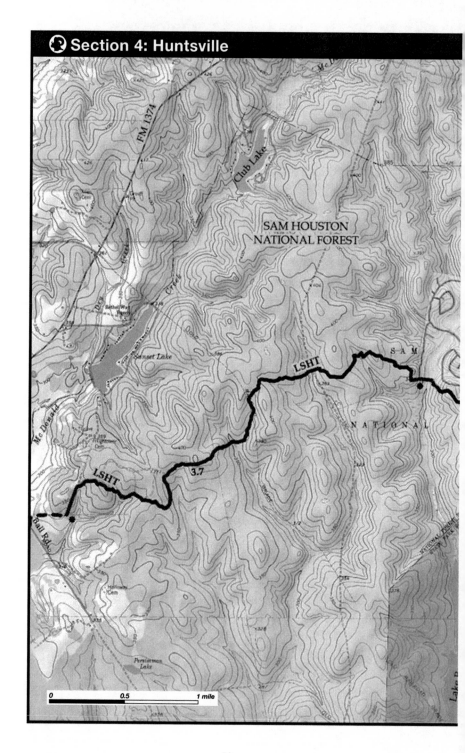

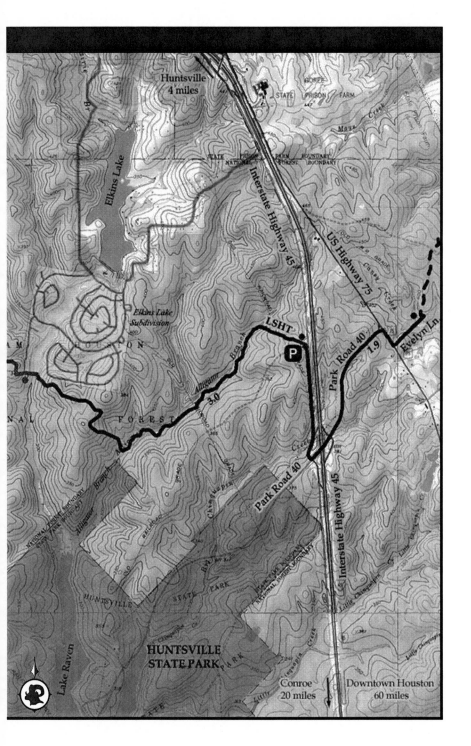

There is also no parking area on Evelyn Lane at the east end of Section 4 at LSHT mile 36.9.

There is no official parking lot or trailhead in Elkins Lake Subdivision, but a car could be parked in the neighborhood for dayhikes. To access the LSHT at mile 32 where it crosses through the outskirts of the Elkins Lake Subdivision, from the I-45 feeder road about 5 miles south the city of Huntsville, or about 2 miles north of the Huntsville State Park exit off of I-45, turn onto Augusta Drive headed west into the Elkins Lake Subdivision. Go 0.5 mile to the intersection of Augusta with Greenbriar Street. Turn left on Greenbriar and go 1.1 miles to River Oaks Drive. Turn right onto River Oaks Drive, then left on West Green Briar Drive, and then veer left onto Camelia Drive. Camelia ends at a circular drive where you will see a small road at the head of the circle.

To get to the LSHT, you'll either drive or walk a few feet up this small drive and turn right on the un-striped, paved road that leads to the water treatment facility. Just after you cross the cattle grate, you'll see the LSHT heading off into the woods westbound. The eastbound LSHT follows the unstriped road you just came up and crosses over the Camelia Lake spillway.

The only official parking lot in Section 4 is along the LSHT at mile 35 where the LSHT Huntsville Trailhead Parking Lot #7 is located on the west side of I-45 along the two-way feeder road adjacent to the interstate. There is no potable water here, but Huntsville State Park, which has some, is about 2 miles south of this parking lot. LSHT Parking Lot #7 is a little smaller than the other official lots; it is well-signed and visible from the road.

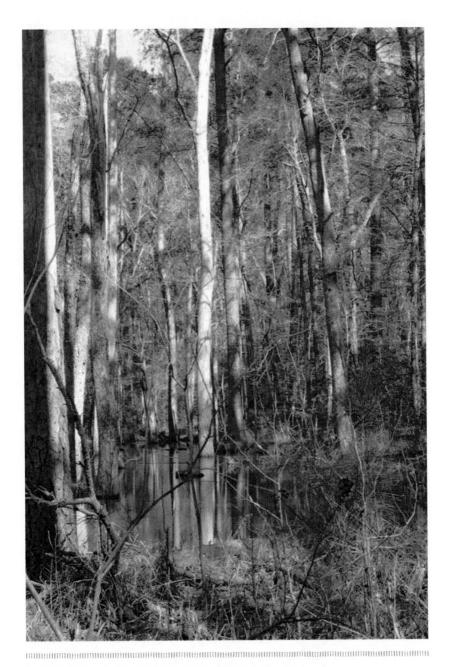

A beautiful swamp at mile 33.1 near Alligator Branch

SECTION 4 GPS Waypoints	
End of Cotton Creek Cemetery Road at LSHT mile 28.3	N 30°38.082' W 95°34.964'
Camelia Lake Spillway	N 30°38.848' W 95°32.505'
LSHT Huntsville Trailhead Parking Lot #7 along Interstate 45	N 30°38.995' W 95°30.636'
Turn under I-45 onto Park Road 40	N 30°38.372' W 95°30.600'
Junction of Park Road 40 and Highway 75	N 30°39.101' W 95°30.127'
End of road walk on Evelyn Lane at mile 37	N 30°39.172' W 95°29.833'

SUPPLIES AND ACCOMMODATIONS

Huntsville State Park, located near the east end of Section 4, offers a good stopover within walking distance of the LSHT that will appeal to thru-hikers. To reach the park, turn east (right if you are on the LSHT road walk headed south along the I-45 feeder road) onto Park Road 40 at the intersection of the I-45 feeder road and Park Road 40 at LSHT mile 35.6 (instead of turning left to follow the LSHT road walk) and go about 1 mile to reach the park entry gate ($4 entrance fee).

Farther into the park (another 0.5 to 1 mile), there are developed campgrounds (fee of $12 per campsite per night for hikers) with potable water, restrooms with running water and hot showers, pay phones, vending machines, a seasonal camp store, and boat rentals. For those interested in overnight parking, there is a $5 fee per vehicle per day (ask the park about other parking restrictions). Upon check-in at the entrance gate, be sure to ask for a map of the park. The park's camp store is seasonal and has limited supplies, so if you need food, you may want to call the park ahead of time to see if you can mail food to yourself in care of the park staff before you begin your hike.

Huntsville (population: 37,537), one of Texas's oldest towns, is located approximately 6 miles north of LSHT Trailhead Parking Lot #7. Of course, a town this size has nearly every accommodation or resupply option a hiker could need. Huntsville also hosts several interesting attractions, including the Sam Houston Homestead and Memorial Museum, the Sam Houston Statue and Visitor's Center, and the Prison Museum.

The following are the services closest to the LSHT: It is 2 miles north from where you come out at the trailhead on I-45 to a combination Citgo convenience store and gas station (on the feeder road). It is 4.5 miles north from the trailhead to a large freeway exit (at FM 1374 East) where there is the Sam Houston Daily Rate Extended Stay Hotel, Country Inn Steak and Seafood Restaurant, Dairy Queen, Super 8 Motel, Gateway Inn and Suites, and three gas stations with ATMs. Continue north following signs to reach the main area of the town of Huntsville (downtown is at the intersection of Highways 75 and 30 about 6 miles north of LSHT Trailhead Parking Lot #7) if you need further services.

The town of New Waverly (population: 950) is approximately 8 miles south of the intersection of Park Road 40 and Highway 75 (on Highway 75). New Waverly does not offer any overnight lodging, but does have several combination gas station and convenience stores, restaurants, an auto parts store, a library, and a grocery store.

WATER

Two reliable water sources grace Section 4: a fairly clear, wild pond at mile 28.9 and the large, clear waters of Alligator Branch between miles 33.3 and 34.3 (access to the creek is easiest at mile 33.3). Camelia Lake, crossed midway through this section at mile 32.1, is not recommended as a water source due to constant runoff from the lawns and streets that surround it. A 1-mile detour at LSHT mile 35.6 (right onto Park Road 40) will bring the hiker to the entrance gate of Huntsville State Park where potable water (and cold soda in vending machines) is available.

TRAIL DESCRIPTION

As Cotton Creek Cemetery Road transitions into an even smaller dirt road and enters the Sam Houston National Forest at LSHT mile 28.4, you enter Section 4. Follow this old dirt road to an intersection with a very small logging track on the right at mile 28.8. Turn right, walking over a dirt mound, and follow the LSHT trail markers into the woods. (Remember that if you are westbound, you need to reverse all directions, left and right, in these

A lovely trailside pond in the Huntsville Section at mile 28.4

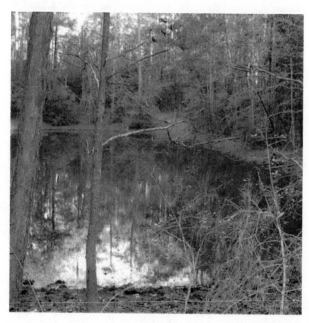

trail descriptions.) Soon, you discover a pond filled with green water that offers a few campsites ▲ and an acceptable water source for those carrying water filters. **MILE MARKER 29** is reached just after the pond.

▲ **Campsite**

At mile 29.4, the sharp-eyed hiker may spot an eight-foot-high game fence that parallels the LSHT on the right through the trees. Cross a seasonal drainage and watch for wooden milepost 29, which is located at contemporary mile 29.5. You may notice a few large oaks and pine trees nearby. Just after crossing a pipeline right-of-way where the game fence is clearly in view to the right, you'll pass **MILE MARKER 30**. This opening could make a sunny, but waterless, camp. ▲ An old hiker gate at a fence line at mile 30.2 presents no obstacle nowadays, but as you near mile 30.4, heavy brush may begin to close in on the trail. A tornado passed through this area several years ago, leaving openings in the tree canopy where mature trees were knocked down by high winds. This is one way that nature gives young plants and trees a chance to grow in thick forests. Watch for Southern red cedar and American holly in this area.

▲ **Campsite**

Don't miss the left turn at mile 30.6. Follow an old barbed wire fence line on a pine-needle-covered trail that makes for more open, pleasant walking. In fact, waterless camping ▲ could be made on either side of the trail at mile 30.7. Watch for **MILE MARKER 31** between the crossings of two seasonal drainages just prior to arriving at another, brushier pipeline right-of-way. At mile 31.3, among old pine trees, you may pick up the sounds of the Elkins Lake Subdivision water treatment facility. It is hidden by the trees, but can be noisy. The small stream you pass at mile 31.5 may be flowing, but its vicinity to the water treatment plant makes it a suspect water source. This area is also frequented by feral pigs; evidence of their presence can be seen along the

▲ **Campsite**

sides of the trail as rooted-up clumps of dirt and plant matter, as well as occasional mud wallows.

Cross another seasonal drainage before spotting an old wooden milepost. Climb a knoll under big trees, and finally spot several houses in Elkins Lake Subdivision at mile 31.9. Another 50 yards of walking brings you to MILE MARKER 32 and, soon after, a small road. Turn left on this unstriped, paved road (the water treatment facility is down this road to the right). Walk on the road downhill toward the lake and over a cattle grate. You have now reached an interesting hiker obstacle: the Camelia Lake Dam. The LSHT crosses directly over the dam where water trickles across a mossy flat spillway. This spillway can be very slippery, so take your time crossing it. (There is no better way to continue on the LSHT without walking through the neigh-

Crossing the Camelia Lake spillway

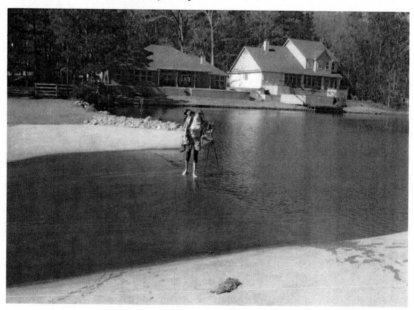

borhood's confusing streets or fording the stream in the thick woods below the spillway.)

After crossing the spillway, head up the rise through the hiker gates. Veer to the right after the second hiker gate and walk over a dirt hump intended to keep ATVs and bikes off of the trail. Continue directly into the woods; do not continue into the neighborhood. It is in everyone's best interest if you do not linger or trespass on anyone's home site or property here. Continued local support for the LSHT relies on hikers respectfully crossing through privately owned areas such as Elkins Lake Subdivision. For this reason, never rely on this neighborhood as a source of trail information or water. Come prepared with your own resources; filtering water out of Camelia Lake—because of local yard and street pollution—is not a good option.

The LSHT heads uphill after leaving Camelia Lake as it begins a 3-mile stretch of uninterrupted woods before reaching I-45. You may continue to see houses and hear dogs to the left of the trail for the next half mile. The first waterless campsites ▲ can be found at mile 32.6 in an open forest of mature pines. Continue to follow a pretty ridge rich in upland hardwood species, such as sassafras, flowering dogwood, rusty blackhaw, and post oak mixed with loblolly and shortleaf pine. After passing **MILE MARKER 33**, the trail heads downhill into the bottomlands of Alligator Branch, a fairly large creek. On quiet days, beautifully colored wood ducks may be resident in the swamps that you'll cross at mile 33.1. Expect to get your feet very muddy, if not soaked, for a short stretch. And watch for trees ringed at the base by busy beavers, animals that were all but extinct in this region 30 years ago.

Alligator Branch flows year-round with clear water over pure white sands that are common along

▲ **Campsite**

the larger waterways of East Texas. In warmer months, you may even discover a small swimming (or at least soaking) hole along this fine creek. Despite its name, it is very doubtful that you will spot an American alligator here, though this is one of the finest sections of the LSHT for bird-watching. At mile 33.3, there is a pretty spot under the canopy of a holly growing on the creek bank, one of the best places to collect water if you need it. Small natural clearings along the creek allow a small campsite to be made, certainly the best camping to be had until you reenter the woods after the I-45 road walk. Continue to parallel Alligator Branch, passing several isolated oxbows filled with brown, swampy water that serve as important refuges for seasonal waterfowl.

Pass the old wooden milepost 33 at present-day mile 33.7. You may begin to hear the distant roar of the interstate. At mile 33.8, cross up and over an old railroad bed that probably served logging activity in the past. Just before passing **MILE MARKER 34**, the LSHT rejoins Alligator Branch whose banks have now grown quite steep and high. Look for the mottled white bark of sycamore trees adjacent to the trail through this area. Cross a deep V-notched ravine on a footbridge at mile 34.6. Veer to the right at the trail junction at mile 34.8; westbound hikers should watch carefully here, as there are few trail markers in sight. **MILE MARKER 35** is reached just before the trail leaves the woods and enters the LSHT Huntsville Trailhead Parking Lot #7 located on the I-45 feeder road.

Now begin a 2-mile road walk that takes you under I-45 and back to public lands where the LSHT runs on toward Cleveland: from the LSHT Trailhead Parking Lot #7, turn right on the feeder road alongside I-45 for 0.6 mile to a stop sign. Turn left at the stop sign onto Park Road 40 that leads underneath the freeway. (If you turn right here, it is a little over 1 mile along the park road before you reach the entrance to Huntsville State Park, beyond which is developed camping, a small seasonal camp store, potable water, vending machines, and hot showers; entrance and camping fees are required.) Walk under the overpass and continue straight on Park Road 40 for 1.0 mile to a stop sign, passing **MILE MARKER 36** somewhere along the way.

At the stop sign, turn right on Highway 75 and walk 0.1 mile to Evelyn Lane, a smaller road on the left. Turn left onto unstriped, paved Evelyn Lane. Walk past a house with a pond and fence on the left and proceed 0.2 mile to a gated driveway. Just to the right of the blue metal gate (on the left side of Evelyn Lane), near a barbed wire fence, the LSHT heads into the woods with plenty of trail markers showing the way. As you enter the woods, you are between LSHT miles 36.9 and 37.0.

SECTION 4 MILEAGE

MILES W→E	TRAIL POINT	MILES E→W	NOTES
28.3	National forest property boundary; swing to left on old dirt road	67.8	
28.4	Leave old dirt road; turn right over hump into woods on LSHT	67.7	
28.9	Pond	67.2	🚰 ▲
29.0	**MILE MARKER 29**	67.1	
29.5	Seasonal drainage; old wooden milepost 29; turn right	66.6	
30.0	Cross pipeline right-of-way; **MILE MARKER 30**	66.1	▲
30.1	Seasonal drainage	66.0	
30.2	Cross old fence line and hiker gate	65.9	
30.7	Enter open area with potential camping; seasonal drainage	65.4	▲
31.0	Seasonal drainage; **MILE MARKER 31;** large clearing	65.1	
31.3	Elkins Lake Subdivision water treatment plant visible	64.8	
31.5	Seasonal stream	64.6	

SECTION 4 MILEAGE

MILES W→E	TRAIL POINT	MILES E→W	NOTES
32.0	**MILE MARKER 32;** Elkins Lake Subdivision; turn left on paved road	64.1	▬
32.1	Cross Camelia Lake spillway	64.0	
32.6	Seasonal drainage; potential waterless campsites in pine forest	63.5	▲
33.0	**MILE MARKER 33**	63.1	
33.1	Cross tributary of Alligator Branch; swamps	63.0	
33.3	Alligator Branch	62.8	🚰 ▲
33.7	Old wooden milepost 33	62.4	
33.8	Cross old railroad bed	62.3	
34.0	**MILE MARKER 34**	62.1	
34.8	Junction of trails; turn right to follow LSHT	61.3	
35.0	**MILE MARKER 35;** Interstate 45; LSHT Huntsville Trailhead Parking Lot #7; turn right on I-45 feeder road	61.1	▬ 🅿
35.6	Turn left on Park Road 40 and continue under I-45 (Huntsville State Park is approximately 1 mile to the right on Park Road 40)	60.5	▬
36.0	**MILE MARKER 36** on Park Road 40	60.1	
36.6	Turn right onto Highway 75	59.5	▬
36.7	Turn left onto Evelyn Lane	59.4	▬
36.9	Turn left onto LSHT right of blue metal gate in woods	59.2	

MILEAGE CHART KEY

🚰 Water source

🚐 Developed campground

🅿 Parking area/trailhead

▲ Undeveloped campsite or potential camping area

▬ Major roads (jeep tracks and logging roads are not indicated)

Evelyn Lane to Four Notch Trailhead on Forest Service Road 213

OVERVIEW

Only 4.8 miles of Section 5 are routed in the woods. However, the remaining 3.4 miles of road walk are mostly enjoyable, as they follow the scenic country lane named Four Notch Road. Water can be an issue for long-distance or overnight hikers through this section, but the flip side of that concern is a trail nearly free of the intermittent mud and standing water that can be a hindrance in other sections. In the few places where leaves or brush have obscured the trail, the LSHT remains well marked by the aluminum blazes at eye level on trees adjacent to the path. A subtle transition from thick piney woods and swampy bottomlands to more open pine-oak highlands occurs as the LSHT reaches the eastern half of Section 5. Tree species, such as Southern magnolia, not found much to the west of Section 5, are seen in the Phelps Section.

TRAIL ACCESS AND PARKING

There is no parking area on Evelyn Lane at the west end of Section 5 at LSHT mile 36.9. One official parking lot serves Section 5: LSHT Four Notch Trailhead Parking Lot #8 is located at mile 45.1 at the east end of Section 5 on Forest Service (FS) Road 213 0.2 mile off of Four Notch Road. There is no potable water at this large lot, but there is a covered picnic pavilion and trash dumpster. To reach it from the intersection of Highway 75 and Farm to Market (FM) 2296 about 5 miles north of New Waverly, go north for 4.2 miles on FM 2296, then turn east (right) for 2.3 miles on Four Notch Road. At FS 213,

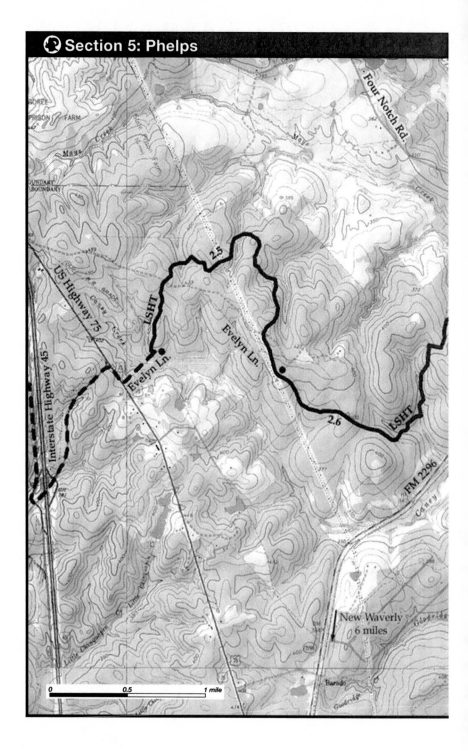

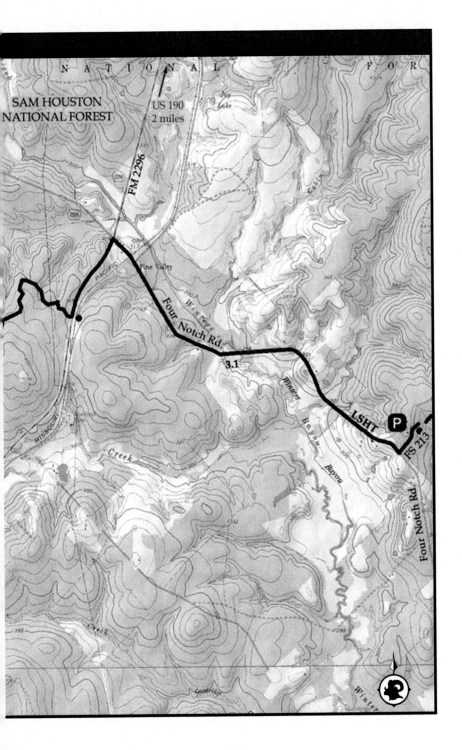

SAM HOUSTON
NATIONAL FOREST

N A T I O N A L

F O R

US 190
2 miles

FM 2296

Pine Valley

PACIFIC

Four Notch Rd.

3.1

Winters

Winters

Bayou

Bayou

MISSOURI

Creek

LSHT

P

FS 213

Four Notch Rd.

Creek

Winters

go north (left) for 0.2 mile to reach the Four Notch parking lot and trailhead at LSHT mile 45.1.

SECTION 5 GPS Waypoints	
End of road walk on Evelyn Lane at mile 37	N 30°39.172' W 95°29.833'
FM 2296 at LSHT mile 42.0	N 30°39.359' W 95°27.547'
Intersection of FM 2296 and Four Notch Road at mile 42.6	N 30°39.765' W 95°27.262'
LSHT Four Notch Trailhead Parking Lot #8 at mile 45.1	N 30°38.769' W 95°25.396

SUPPLIES AND ACCOMMODATIONS

The city of Huntsville and the town of New Waverly, both at the west end of Section 5, offer resupply within a reasonable distance of the LSHT. Only Huntsville offers overnight lodging. See Section 4 (page 71). The east end of Section 5 along Four Notch Road at LSHT Trailhead Parking Lot #8 is a remote area; no supplies or accommodations are located near the trail.

WATER

Unfortunately, Section 5 is one of the driest on the LSHT. In rainy periods or prolonged wet seasons, there are several seasonal drainages throughout this section that may harbor trailside water. However, in most normal to dry seasons, you should plan carefully to carry all the water you need to traverse this section. Along the road walk on Four Notch Road between miles 42.6 and 45.1, there are two creeks, one of which is the large and reliable Winters Bayou. Their proximity to the road and local farms may deter hikers.

TRAIL DESCRIPTION

As you leave Evelyn Lane and the 2-mile road walk at the end of Section 4, the LSHT heads back into the woods just to the right of a blue metal gate near a barbed wire fence and quickly passes **MILE MARKER 37**. At mile 37.4, cross a small seasonal drainage and an old abandoned logging road. Old wooden milepost 37 is located at present-day mile 37.6 just before a large, sandy-bottomed gully. The trail crosses another steep-sided seasonal drainage, traverses through a young pine forest, and begins to zigzag to the right and left before crossing a good jeep road. (Remember that if you are westbound, you need to reverse all directions, left and right, in these trail descriptions.) You may see evidence of past tornado damage here.

In an open grassy area beneath mature pine trees, pass **MILE MARKER 38** just before reaching a utilities right-of-way. A waterless camp ▲ could be made ▲ **Campsite** here. Cross on a small hiker bridge a creek that may harbor a trickle or a puddle at mile 38.2. Ascend a hill and cross a grassy logging road and old wooden milepost 38 at current mile 38.6. Another seasonal drainage follows soon after. Watch for the numerous holly trees that grow to the right of the trail in this area, which feels as if it is seldom walked. There's even a good (waterless) campsite ▲ under a holly on the ▲ **Campsite** left at mile 38.9. Pass **MILE MARKER 39** a few minutes before you reach a jeep track and cross under a power line. Follow the jeep track a little to the left and look for trail markers on the trees; tall grass often obscures the LSHT's entry back into the woods. Enter an area of shortleaf pine and large hardwood trees, including white oak, Southern red oak, black hickory, and sassafras. This is a nice spot for a break.

At mile 39.4, pass through a hiker gate and turn left onto a gravel road near the power lines. This is actually Evelyn Lane again, though it is dirt here. Walk on this road until mile 39.7 where you turn left back into the woods by a hiker sign and a house where dogs may be running loose. As you reenter the peace of the woods, the LSHT passes through a young pine forest along a wide corridor. Just after an old logging road, pass **MILE MARKER 40**. A nice bridge spans a creek that usually has water running in it at mile 40.4. Watch for large white oaks through here, long-lived trees that produce valuable wood often used for making furniture. A large creek at mile 40.5 may also contain water in wet seasons. Cross another seasonal creek, pass **MILE MARKER 41**, enter a mature open pine forest, and then cross a large gravel road at mile 41.2. Eastbound hikers pass one of the first noticeable evergreen Southern magnolia trees (*Magnolia grandiflora*) on the left. Also called the bull bay, its large, thick fragrant blossoms evolved before bees existed and are designed to be pollinated by beetles.

You may notice some "selective logging" activity at mile 41.3. Cross an old logging road at mile 41.6, followed by a seasonal drainage at mile 41.7 and pipeline right-of-way at mile 41.9. The trail may be hard to see underfoot as you near **MILE MARKER 42**, so watch for the well-spaced trail markers in the trees at eye level. However, don't forget to look down occasionally; beautiful mushrooms, such as cinnabar chanterelles, are commonly seen alongside the trail here. You may also notice some houses off to the left. Here, you reach FM 2296 and turn left onto this highway for about a half mile. Reach signed Four Notch Road at mile 42.6 and take a right on this unstriped, paved road, which is directly across from the intersection of the larger FM 2929 with FM 2296. At mile 42.8, cross the railroad tracks and continue straight ahead. Some older LSHT guides describe this road as dirt, but it is now paved. You soon cross a creek that should have running water in it; if you are in need of water, follow this creek a little upstream and off the road to find a good place to collect and treat drinking water. **MILE MARKER 43** is visible along the road in a tree.

At mile 43.7, you pass a house where some large farm dogs may come out to bark at you. Another large creek with running water, Winters Bayou, is crossed on a bridge at mile 43.7. Again, you may be thirsty enough to search for a good place to filter water here. **MILE MARKER 44** is not easily seen but is passed as you come up a hill and follow a curve in the road. Open farmland allows the eye to roam on either side of this little country lane. Except for the occasional dog or two, this is a peaceful, scenic road walk. At mile 44.9, a double-blazed set of trail markers directs you to turn left down dirt FS 213. **MILE MARKER 45** is not visible, but you'll know you've just passed it when you arrive at the oversized parking lot at the end of this section at mile 45.1. This is LSHT Four Notch Trailhead Parking Lot #8. Park service dumpsters, a picnic shelter, and a trailhead bulletin

The winter branches of hardwood trees overhead in the Phelps Section

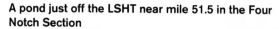

A pond just off the LSHT near mile 51.5 in the Four
Notch Section

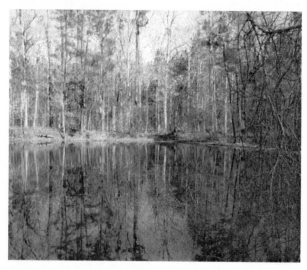

board are located at this wayside. There is no potable
water available. This site is the location of the old Four
Notch fire tower; you may see some of its foundation.
As you leave this parking lot and reenter the woods, the
Phelps road walk ends and you enter Section 6.

SECTION 5 MILEAGE			
MILES W→E	TRAIL POINT	MILES E→W	NOTES
36.9	Turn left into woods right of blue metal gate on Evelyn Lane	59.2	✖
37.0	**MILE MARKER 37**	59.1	
37.4	Seasonal drainage; abandoned logging road	58.7	
37.6	Old wooden milepost 37; large sandy-bottomed gully	58.5	
37.7	Steep-sided seasonal drainage	58.4	
37.8	Jeep track	58.3	
38.0	**MILE MARKER 38** in open grassy area; potential campsite	58.1	▲
38.2	Bridge over small seasonal creek (stagnant water)	57.9	
38.4	Grass-covered logging road	57.7	
38.6	Old wooden milepost 38	57.5	

SECTION 5 MILEAGE

MILES W→E	TRAIL POINT	MILES E→W	NOTES
38.7	Seasonal drainage	57.4	
38.9	Potential campsite under holly tree on left	57.2	▲
39.0	**MILE MARKER 39**	57.1	
39.1	Follow jeep track left across power line	57.0	
39.4	Hiker gate; left onto gravel road (Evelyn Lane)	56.7	▭
39.7	Reenter woods on left	56.4	
40.0	Old logging road; **MILE MARKER 40**	56.1	
40.4	Bridged seasonal creek (small amount of flowing water)	55.7	
40.5	Large seasonal creek (stagnant water)	55.6	
40.6	Seasonal creek	55.5	
41.0	**MILE MARKER 41**	55.1	
41.2	Gravel road	54.9	
41.6	Old logging road	54.5	
41.7	Seasonal drainage	54.4	
41.9	Pipeline crossing	54.2	
42.0	**MILE MARKER 42;** left onto FM 2296	54.1	▭
42.6	Right onto unstriped, paved Four Notch Road	53.5	▭
42.8	Cross railroad tracks; continue on Four Notch Road	53.3	
43.0	Creek (low volume); **MILE MARKER 43** along Four Notch Road	53.1	🚰 *
43.7	Cross Winters Bayou on Four Notch Road bridge (high volume)	52.4	🚰
44.0	**MILE MARKER 44** on Four Notch Road	52.1	
44.9	Left onto dirt FS 213	51.2	▭
45.0	**MILE MARKER 45** on FS 213	51.1	
45.1	LSHT Four Notch Trailhead Parking Lot #8; reenter woods on right	51.0	▭ 🅿

Water here is seasonal and dependent on weather conditions.

MILEAGE CHART KEY

🚰	Water source	▲	Undeveloped campsite or potential camping area
🚐	Developed campground		
🅿	Parking area/trailhead	▭▭	Major roads (jeep tracks and logging roads are not indicated)

Four Notch Road to Junction of
Forest Service Roads 207 and 202

OVERVIEW

The Four Notch Loop area was devastated by a pine bark beetle infestation in the early 1980s. The U.S. Forest Service cut, burned, and replanted the damaged forests between 1982 and 1987. The observant hiker will be able to discern where natural, wild forest transitions to the replanted areas, which are now covered in dense vegetation. Despite the large segments of new growth, this section still retains a wild, remote feel and a diversity of forest types. The 10-mile, well-maintained Four Notch Loop Trail, of which the main LSHT is a part, offers an excellent opportunity for weekend loop hikes with easy trail access at LSHT Trailhead Parking Lot #8. Boswell Creek is located in a beautiful hardwood bottomland and is large enough to offer swimming holes. In most seasons, it's easy to find a place to hop from one sandy bank to another; however, this creek can present an insurmountable obstacle during heavy rains. The Four Notch Section is popular with Boy Scouts and other hiking groups, but there is plenty of space for everyone in its wilderness.

TRAIL ACCESS AND PARKING

To reach the LSHT Trailhead Parking Lot #8 at the west end of Section 6 (LSHT mile 45.1) from the intersection of Highway 75 and Farm to Market (FM) 2296 about 5 miles north of New Waverly, go north for 4.2 miles on FM 2296, then turn east (right) for 2.3 miles on Four Notch Road. At Forest Service (FS) Road 213, go north (left) 0.2 mile to reach the Four Notch parking lot and trailhead at LSHT mile 45.1. Trash dumpsters and a covered picnic pavilion are available, but there is no water at this trailhead.

To reach the east end of Section 6 at the junction of Forest Service (FS) Roads 207 and 202 (LSHT mile 54.4), proceed to the tiny hamlet of Evergreen at the intersection of Farm to Market (FM) 945 and Highway 150, about 15 miles east of New Waverly. From this intersection in Evergreen, head west (toward New Waverly) for 0.25 mile and turn right onto John Warren Road (FS 202). Follow FS 202 for approximately 7.5 miles until you reach the intersection with FS 207. The LSHT enters the woods on the right of the road where these two dirt roads intersect. There is room to park here, though it is not an official (improved) parking area. As with nearly every parking area on the LSHT, no water is available.

SECTION 6 GPS Waypoints	
LSHT Four Notch Trailhead Parking Lot #8 at LSHT mile 45.1	N 30°38.769' W 95°25.396'
West junction with Four Notch Loop Trail	N 30°38.837' W 95°25.117'
Boswell Creek at LSHT mile 48.2	N 30°38.085' W 95°24.219'
East junction with Four Notch Loop Trail	N 30°39.220' W 95°23.016'
Intersection of FS 207 and FS 202 at mile 54.4	N 30°37.999' W 95°19.172'

SUPPLIES AND ACCOMMODATIONS

Both the west and east ends of Section 6 are located in remote areas. The town of New Waverly (population: 950) is 5 miles north of the intersection of Highway 75 and FM 2296. New Waverly does not offer any overnight lodging, but does offer several combination gas station and convenience stores, restaurants, a post office, an auto parts store, a library, and a grocery store. The closest overnight accommodations, as well as a

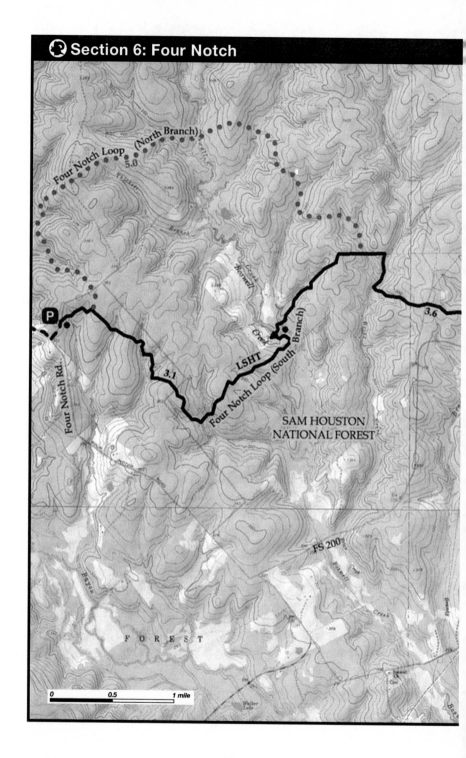

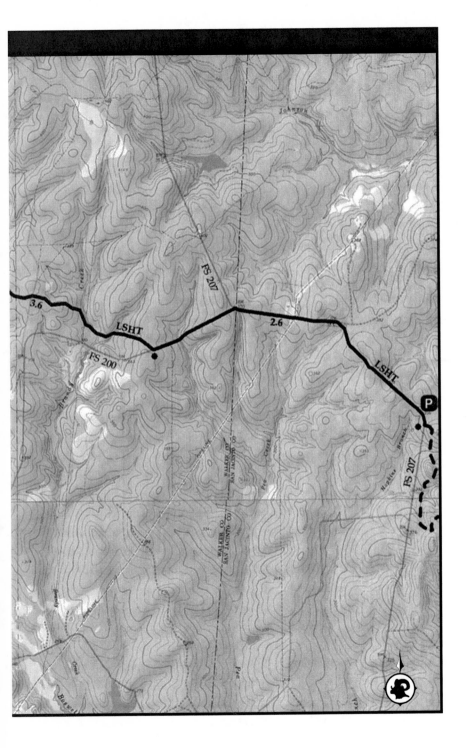

large selection of other services, can be found along Interstate 45 in and around the town of Huntsville (see Section 4, page 71, for more information).

WATER

Unlike the Phelps Section, the Four Notch Section is blessed with abundant water sources. Overnight hikers should be able to camp near water at Boswell Creek or at the wild pond at mile 51.5. In wet periods, the seasonal creeks also harbor water. Due to the sandy soils in this region, the creeks tend to run clear, not muddy.

TRAIL DESCRIPTION

From the LSHT Four Notch Trailhead Parking Lot #8, head into the woods following the trail and LSHT markers visible on the right as you entered the parking lot at mile 45.1. (Remember that if you are westbound, you need to reverse all directions, left and right, in these trail descriptions.) After crossing a small seasonal drainage, you soon reach the signed junction of the LSHT and Four Notch Loop Trail at mile 45.4. The loop heads off to the left following red-striped trail markers, while the main LSHT turns right. Although this description focuses on the main route, feel free to follow either branch, as they meet again 4 miles down the main branch (the left-hand fork offers great hiking through some of the most beautiful forests on the LSHT, also crosses Boswell Creek, and is a little longer—closer to 6 miles—before it meets up with the main LSHT).

At mile 45.7, cross a deep drainage that may harbor a trickle or a stagnant pool, followed quickly by a logging road. You may spot some large black tupelo (blackgum) trees, as well as Southern magnolia, a tree that is much more common on the eastern half of the LSHT. Another usually dry, steep-banked creek is crossed at mile 45.9. The trail intersects and briefly follows a faint logging road just before reaching **MILE MARKER 46**. In the next half mile, you cross several seasonal drainages before reaching a large open area near a dirt road. Although there is room for several tents here, ▲ beware that this site is usually littered with trash and can attract car campers and hunters. As you pass the campfire pit, hang a right onto a wide path. Reach a good dirt road, jog slightly to the left, and proceed through an opening that looks like an impromptu parking spot. Continue straight ahead following trail markers.

▲ **Campsite**

A more secluded (but waterless) camping spot ▲ is found on the right at mile 46.7. Several of the typical seasonal creeks are crossed, including one at **MILE MARKER 47**. A few large oaks grow in this hardwood forest. Two old logging roads are crossed (take a sharp left on the first one) before reaching a big open flat at mile 47.4 where several tents could be set up (of course, it's also waterless). ▲ At mile 47.5, you join up with the old logging road again and follow it for some time. More waterless camping ▲ could be made at mile 47.6 just before the old road splits (follow the left fork). Cross a seasonal creek and follow the road as it jogs to the left and then meets another old road. At **MILE MARKER 48**, thru-hikers may want to pause and reflect on reaching the LSHT's halfway point.

▲ **Campsite**

▲ **Campsite**

▲ **Campsite**

Young pine forests give way to a beautiful hardwood bottomland. Beaver activity is evident all along Boswell Creek's banks, which you reach at mile 48.2. Good backcountry campsites ▲ are found throughout the woods in this area. The creek's clear waters flow year-round and offer a good water source. In fact, you may spot fish in its waters. Frequent flooding has washed out

▲ **Campsite**

all hiker bridges over Boswell Creek, so hikers are left to find their own way across the creek. In normal to dry seasons, the ford should be a quick hop across. However, if it has been raining heavily, *this high-banked creek may be extremely hazardous to cross.* Turn back if you find conditions too dangerous for a ford.

After you cross Boswell Creek, turn right and follow it for a short stroll before turning and heading off into the woods. Cross a tributary of the creek near an old deer blind in a tree. At mile 48.5, a fence becomes visible on the left. After crossing yet another seasonal drainage and passing **MILE MARKER 49**, intersect the Four Notch Loop Trail at its east end at LSHT mile 49.4 at a well-signed junction. This junction offers a nice spot to rest or eat lunch, surrounded by upland hardwood forest dominated by white oak and winged elms. About 40 yards southeast of this junction is a natural pond where you can see large black tupelo and palmettos. Cross a small drainage and traverse a noticeable rise in the land.

At mile 49.7, you meet up with and follow Briar Creek, a large creek (usually running with clear water) that is bridged at mile 49.9. Pass **MILE MARKER 50**, cross a small seasonal drainage among red maples, and then cross FS 206 (a good dirt road). There is some informal parking on either side of the road here. The trail through this area is sometimes open but usually brushy, and like the past few miles, it may sometimes be necessary to use the trail markers for visual navigation as you walk.

Just before a pipeline right-of-way, pass **MILE MARKER 51**. Oaks and mature pine trees mix throughout this riparian woodland, making a pleasant spot for a break. After crossing several seasonal drainages, reach a pond on the left at mile 51.5. Though it can

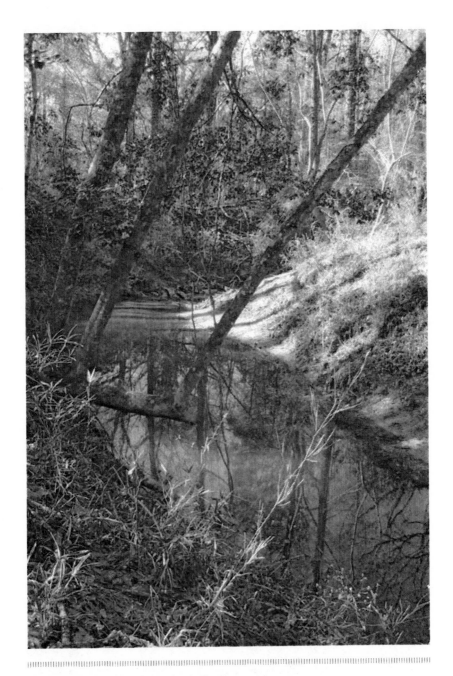

Boswell Creek in the Four Notch Section

be a picturesque spot in the fall, briars and brush can

Campsite ▲ make finding a good campsite ▲ near the pond challenging. The waters in the pond are colored like strong tea by tannins, natural chemical substances (harmless to ingest in small quantities) that leach into the water from leaves and pine needles. You may find that the water in this pond is not as clear and appealing as that in the trailside pond in the Huntsville Section.

Cross an old logging road at mile 51.7 that offers a grassy clearing for campers but is close to FS 200. When you reach this gravel road, turn left and follow it for 0.7 mile. Along the way, pass a fairly large creek that should harbor running water and pass **MILE MARKER 52** (LSHT mile markers 52, 53, and 54 may not be visible along the road walk). At mile 52.4, reach a stop sign and turn right onto FS 207, which is also a good gravel road. Walk past a gas processing plant at

Poisonous *Amanita muscaria* mushrooms along the LSHT

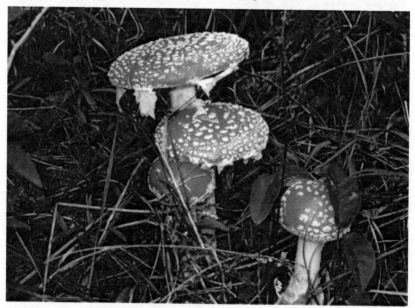

mile 52.9 and along old clear-cuts recently replanted after **MILE MARKER 53**. Continue past a small dirt road that heads off to the left; you curve to the right on the main road. More ugly clear-cuts present themselves as you pass **MILE MARKER 54**.

The junction of FS 207 with FS 202 is located at mile 54.4. Here, where FS 202 branches off to the left, the entry of the LSHT back into the woods is well-signed and easy to see. There is an informal parking area. This is the end of Section 6 and beginning of the seventh section, which is named Big Woods.

SECTION 6 MILEAGE

MILES W→E	TRAIL POINT	MILES E→W	NOTES
45.1	LSHT Four Notch Trailhead Parking Lot #8; reenter woods on right	51.0	⊷ 🅿
45.4	Junction with Four Notch Loop Trail; main LSHT turns right	50.7	
45.7	Deep seasonal drainage; logging road	50.4	
45.9	Seasonal creek	50.2	
46.0	Faint logging road; **MILE MARKER 46**	50.1	
46.2	Seasonal creek	49.9	
46.5	Trash-filled hunter camp on dirt road; potential campsites	49.6	▲
46.7	Potential campsites on right; parallel seasonal drainage on right	49.4	▲
46.8	Large seasonal creek	49.3	
47.0	**MILE MARKER 47**; seasonal creek	49.1	
47.1	Left onto old logging road	49.0	
47.2	Cross logging road	48.9	
47.4	Large open flat; potential camping	48.7	▲
47.5	Right onto old logging road	48.6	
47.6	Large open flat; potential camping; seasonal creek	48.5	▲
47.8	Junction of old logging roads	48.3	
48.0	**MILE MARKER 48**	48.1	
48.2	Boswell Creek; camping (high volume; good water)	47.9	🚰 ▲
48.7	Seasonal drainage	47.4	
49.0	**MILE MARKER 49**	47.1	

SECTION 6 MILEAGE

MILES W→E	TRAIL POINT	MILES E→W	NOTES
49.4	Junction with Four Notch Loop Trail	46.7	
49.5	Small seasonal drainage; hill	46.6	
49.9	Bridge over Briar Creek (low flow; good water)	46.2	💧
50.0	**MILE MARKER 50**	46.1	
50.4	Cross over FS 206	45.7	▬
51.0	**MILE MARKER 51**; pipeline right-of-way	45.1	
51.1	Large seasonal creek	45.0	
51.3	Large seasonal creek	44.8	
51.5	Pond on left; camping (dark tannin-colored water)	44.6	💧 ▲
51.8	Left onto gravel FS 200	44.3	▬
51.9	Creek (low volume; good water) along FS 200	44.2	💧
52.0	**MILE MARKER 52** (not visible on road)	44.1	
52.4	Turn right onto gravel FS 207 at stop sign	43.7	▬
53.0	Gas processing plant; **MILE MARKER 53** (not visible on road)	43.1	
54.0	**MILE MARKER 54** (not visible on road)	42.1	
54.4	Junction of FS 207 and 202; reenter woods	41.7	▬ 🅿

MILEAGE CHART KEY

💧	Water source	▲	Undeveloped campsite or potential camping area
🚐	Developed campground		
🅿	Parking area/trailhead	▬▬	Major roads (jeep tracks and logging roads are not indicated)

Junction of Forest Service Roads 207 and 202 to Ira Denson Road

OVERVIEW

Woods, woods, and more woods! The Big Woods Section lives up to its name, leading the hiker through many uninterrupted miles of typical East Texas forests. These pine and oak forests are riddled by numerous seasonal creeks and fern-lined drainages that feed the watershed of Winters Bayou, itself a major tributary of the San Jacinto River. However, *reliable* water sources are scarce. During warm or dry seasons, hikers should plan to carry in all the water needed for hiking and camping.

Human development is also relatively sparse in the Big Woods Section of the LSHT. The trail skirts private property that abuts the Sam Houston National Forest in a few places. Small scale road-building and logging may be visible in these areas, but no major roads or housing developments are seen anywhere along the 8.4-mile route. No notable trail obstacles are present to the hiker. The extended muddy areas and swamps present in so many of the other sections are nearly absent here.

Creeks and drainages are easy to cross in all but the worst weather conditions. The trail continues to be well marked except for a few short stretches detailed below. Provided hikers are careful to carry in drinking water, Section 7 offers numerous quiet spots to pitch a tent and enjoy the peace of the big woods.

TRAIL ACCESS AND PARKING

To reach the west end of Section 7 at the junction of Forest Service (FS) Roads 207 and 202 (LSHT mile 54.4), proceed to the tiny hamlet of Evergreen at the

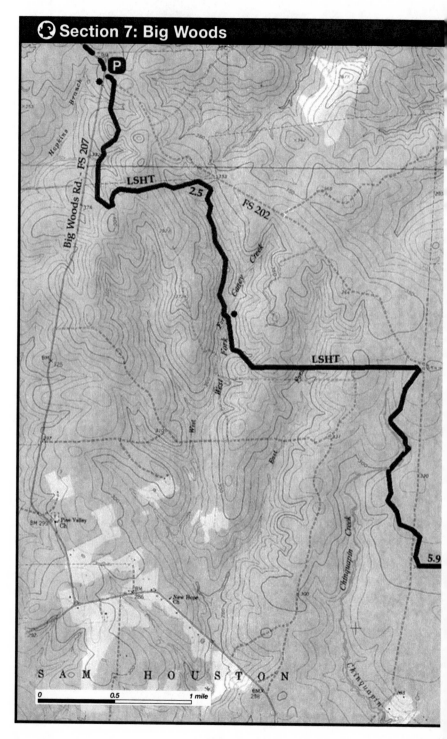

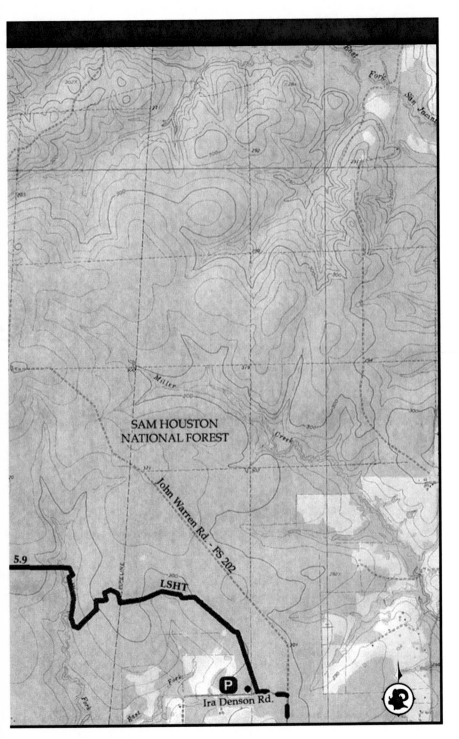

SAM HOUSTON
NATIONAL FOREST

John Warren Rd. - FS 202

5.9

LSHT

P

Ira Denson Rd.

Miller

Creek

Fork

San Jacint

intersection of Farm to Market (FM) 945 and Highway 150, about 15 miles east of New Waverly. From this intersection in Evergreen, head west (toward New Waverly) for 0.25 mile and turn right onto John Warren Road (FS 202). Follow FS 202 for approximately 7.5 miles until you reach the intersection with FS 207. No water or trash disposal is available at this trailhead.

To reach the east end of Section 7 at LSHT Big Woods Trailhead Parking Lot #9 (LSHT mile 62.8), begin from the same intersection of FM 945 and Highway 150 in Evergreen. From this intersection in Evergreen, also head west for 0.25 mile and turn right onto John Warren Road (FS 202). Follow FS 202 for 1.7 miles to the intersection with Ira Denson Road on the left. Take a left onto Ira Denson Road and go 0.2 mile where LSHT Big Woods Trailhead Parking Lot #9 is located on the right side of the road. No water or trash disposal is available at this trailhead.

SECTION 7 GPS Waypoints	
Intersection of FS 207 and FS 202 at mile 54.4	N 30°37.999' W 95°19.172'
West Fork Caney Creek at mile 56.9	N 30°37.258' W 95°18.493'
LSHT Big Woods Trailhead Parking Lot #9 on Ira Denson Road	N 30°34.656' W 95°15.464'

SUPPLIES AND ACCOMMODATIONS

The west end of Section 7 is located in a remote area and, therefore, has no supplies or accommodations nearby. The east end of Section 7 is also remote, but just ahead along the next section's road walk, the hiker passes through Evergreen, a small hamlet of private residences with a vacant store and nonworking phone booth. From Evergreen, it is approximately 9 miles to Coldspring (population: 691) east on Highway 150. Coldspring does not offer any overnight lodging, but does offer a local diner, barbeque restaurant, post office, dollar store, gas stations, and a large grocery store. The larger, full-service town of Shepherd (population: 2,262) along U.S. Highway 59 is 11 miles southeast of Coldspring and offers several motels.

WATER

Section 7 harbors several large intermittent (seasonal) creeks and streams. In dry periods, do *not* expect to find water in this section. Even in wet seasons, if you plan to camp in the Big Woods Section, consider carrying all the water needed to make a waterless camp. The best spot to find water is at the crossing of the West Fork of Caney Creek at mile 56.9.

TRAIL DESCRIPTION

The junction of FS 207 with FS 202 is located at LSHT mile 54.4. Here, where FS 202 branches off to the left, the entry of the LSHT back into the woods is well signed and easy to see. Cross a deep seasonal drainage at mile 54.6 and enter a fairly open area where a waterless camp ▲ could be made to either side of the ▲ **Campsite** trail in a mixed forest. Pass several seasonal drainages before reaching **MILE MARKER 55**. Mile 54 measures, at 1.2 miles, a little too long. This anomaly is probably related to past inaccurate measurement made of the miles along the road walk at the end of Section 6. Despite this inaccuracy, this guidebook describes the LSHT mileage as it relates to the present-day LSHT mile markers to avoid confusion.

Another small drainage is crossed before coming out into an appealing open area in a pine forest. The trail is in good condition as you continue, crossing a twin set of seasonal drainages at mile 55.3. Next, cross an old sunken road and a clearing off to the left where **Campsite** ▲ you could put up a tent. ▲ Recross the old road at mile 55.5 and then cross a seasonal drainage twice at mile 55.8. Just as you reach a drainage on the left, pass **MILE MARKER 56**. (Remember that if you are westbound, you need to reverse all directions, left and right, in these trail descriptions.)

Again, dip into and out of that same seasonal drainage a few more times and begin to parallel it at mile 56.5. This is the intermittent West Fork of Caney Creek, which you eventually cross at mile 56.9 and where you have an opportunity to collect water, if there is any to be had. As you climb out of this drainage, the trail turns alongside a barbed wire fence line on the right. Soon after, reach a marked property boundary where private land abuts national forest. You may see evidence of small scale road-building on the private land along the LSHT here.

Pass **MILE MARKER 57** in a young pine forest where wild pigs often root up the soil along the trail. Cross a U-shaped sandy-bottomed seasonal drainage at mile 57.7 in a pretty area. Just after an uphill jaunt, pass **MILE MARKER 58** in a mixed woodland home to some big oaks. In a pinch, you may be able **Campsite** ▲ to find a small camping spot off to the left here. ▲ Cross an old road bed and then twice cross a steep seasonal drainage filled with ferns at mile 58.2. Cross a recently constructed logging track at mile 58.5 and watch for the giant oak tree to the left of the trail at mile 58.8. You may notice a clear-cut area through the trees nearby and an open area ahead that could do as **Campsite** ▲ a waterless campsite. ▲ Feral pigs often tear up the soils in this area; they are not native to the U.S. but are descendants of domestic pigs escaped or released

from settlements dating back as far as the first Europeans in East Texas.

Pass **MILE MARKER 59** and dip into the seasonal
fern-lined Chinquapin Creek. Enter a young pine forest. You may cross bulldozer tracks at mile 59.4 and
notice an open area at the edge of this forest where
high yellow grass grows conspicuously. Cross a seasonal drainage and then cross a small gravel road at
a right-trending diagonal at mile 59.8. **MILE MARKER 60**
is soon followed by a set of small drainages and an old
logging road where you'll make a left turn. Take care
at mile 60.2 to follow the markers straight ahead; do
not turn onto the old jeep track heading uphill. Cross a
large sandy seasonal creek at mile 60.4. Several smaller
drainages are crossed before reaching a junction of
trails at mile 60.9. Follow the LSHT left and soon pass

A hiker relaxes in camp after a long day on the trail.

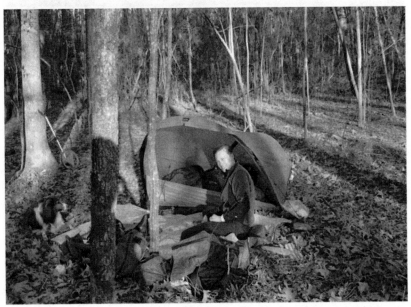

Campsite

MILE MARKER 61. At mile 61.4, reach an open area at a junction of old logging roads where a waterless camp could be made. ▲ Trail markers may be few and far between here. Just keep walking straight ahead, following the trail as it gradually veers right before taking a sharp left at mile 61.5. Reach a rough-looking jungly drainage at mile 61.7. Make a right turn at mile 61.9 to meet up with an old logging track. The trail zigs and zags before passing **MILE MARKER 62.**

Pass a fence corner and post at mile 62.4. More bulldozer activity may be evident around this property boundary off to the right. In a homogenous young pine forest, walk down the wide and pleasant trail to mile 62.8 and the end of Section 7 at LSHT Big Woods Trailhead Parking Lot #9 at dirt Ira Denson Road. Ahead is the beginning of Section 8 and the longest road walk on the LSHT.

SECTION 7 MILEAGE

MILES W→E	TRAIL POINT	MILES E→W	NOTES
54.4	Junction of FS 207 and 202; reenter woods	41.7	▬ 🅿
54.6	Deep seasonal drainage; potential camping	41.5	▲
55.0	Series of seasonal drainages; **MILE MARKER 55**	41.1	
55.3	Set of twin seasonal drainages	40.8	
55.4	Cross sunken road twice; potential campsite	40.7	▲
55.8	Cross seasonal drainage twice (stagnant water)	40.3	
56.0	**MILE MARKER 56**; drainage to the left crossed in 0.1 mile	40.1	
56.2	Seasonal drainage (trickle of water) (West Fork Caney Creek)	39.9	
56.9	West Fork Caney Creek (low volume; clear); property boundary	39.2	⚲ *
57.0	**MILE MARKER 57**	39.1	
57.7	Shallow seasonal drainage; larger U-shaped drainage	38.4	
58.0	**MILE MARKER 58**; potential camping	38.1	▲
58.1	Old road bed	38.0	

SECTION 7 MILEAGE

MILES W→E	TRAIL POINT	MILES E→W	NOTES
58.2	Cross fern-lined seasonal drainage twice	37.9	
58.5	Logging track	37.6	
58.8	Large oak tree; potential campsites	37.3	▲
59.0	**MILE MARKER 59**	37.1	
59.1	Fern-lined seasonal drainage (Chinquapin Creek)	37.0	
59.5	Seasonal drainage	36.6	
59.8	Small gravel road	36.3	
60.0	**MILE MARKER 60;** several small drainages and old logging road	36.1	
60.2	Old jeep track heads uphill to left; follow LSHT straight ahead	35.9	
60.4	Cross large sandy-bottomed intermittent stream	35.7	
60.6	Cross several small seasonal drainages	35.5	
60.9	Junction of trails; follow LSHT left	35.2	
61.0	**MILE MARKER 61**	35.1	
61.4	Open area at junction of logging roads; potential camping; follow LSHT straight and then right	34.7	▲
61.5	Make a sharp left turn	34.6	
61.7	Deep brushy seasonal drainage	34.4	
62.0	**MILE MARKER 62**	34.1	
62.4	Fence post and corner at property boundary	33.7	
62.8	LSHT Big Woods Trailhead Parking Lot #9; follow LSHT left onto dirt Ira Denson Road	33.3	▬ 🅿

* *Water here is seasonal and dependent on weather conditions.*

MILEAGE CHART KEY

🚰	Water source	▲	Undeveloped campsite or potential camping area
🚐	Developed campground		
🅿	Parking area/trailhead	▬▬▬	Major roads (jeep tracks and logging roads are not indicated)

Ira Denson Road to Double Lake Recreation Area

OVERVIEW

The Magnolia Section is long enough to offer a little of everything. The western end consists of a 5-mile road walk on dirt and blacktop roads. Only a short 0.3-mile stretch of the road walk is along a busy highway; the other miles can be sunny but are usually peaceful. The remaining 7 miles of Section 8 meander through a variety of ecosystems. One of the most amazing of these is the large region of mature evergreen Southern magnolia trees that surround the bottomlands of the East Fork of the San Jacinto River. Here, the LSHT hiker may be surprised to find a rolling landscape and a secret nook in the woods where a small waterfall runs during most seasons. This section may throw some other surprises at the hiker if the season has included any recent flooding. Bridges, particularly the one over the East Fork, have been known to wash out. As long as the waterways are not flooded, adventurous hikers can easily ford them if needed.

Double Lake Recreation Area, built in 1937 by the Civilian Conservation Corps, offers several diversions from hiking. This 23-acre spring-fed lake is periodically stocked with bass, bluegill, and catfish. There is even a small sandy beach and swimming area to be enjoyed in warmer months. The LSHT is in good condition through the Magnolia Section with only one noted area where the trail is not well marked. About midway through the section is one of the few primitive backcountry campgrounds built and maintained expressly for LSHT hikers.

TRAIL ACCESS AND PARKING

To reach the west end of Section 8 at LSHT Big Woods Trailhead Parking Lot #9 (LSHT mile 62.8), begin from the intersection of Farm to Market (FM) 945 and Highway 150 in Evergreen. Head west for 0.25 mile and turn right onto John Warren Road (Forest Service [FS] Road 202). Follow FS 202 for 1.7 miles to the intersection with Ira Denson Road on the left. Take a left onto Ira Denson Road and go 0.2 mile where Trailhead Parking Lot #9 is on the right side of the road.

To reach Double Lake Recreation Area, take Highway 150 from Evergreen 5.7 miles east to Farm to Market (FM) 2025 (or 25 miles east from New Waverly). Turn right (south) onto FM 2025 for 0.4 mile and turn left onto Double Lake Park Road. Ask camp hosts about parking a car within the recreation area; there is a $6 fee per day to park here.

SECTION 8 GPS Waypoints	
LSHT Trailhead Parking Lot #9 on Ira Denson Road	N 30°34.656' W 95°15.464'
Intersection of Ira Denson Rd. and FS 202 (John Warren Rd.)	N 30°34.644' W 95°15.281'
Intersection of Hwy. 150 and FM 945 in Evergreen	N 30°33.667' W 95°14.335'
LSHT Trailhead Parking Lot #10 at FM 945 and Butch Arther Rd. (Jacobs Rd.)	N 30°31.666' W 95°13.207'
LSHT Primitive Campsite #2 at LSHT mile 68.6	N 30°31.586' W 95°12.110'
Crossing of the East Fork of the San Jacinto River	N 30°32.045' W 95°11.074'
LSHT Trailhead Parking Lot #11 on FM 2025	N 30°32.886' W 95°08.640'
Double Lake Recreation Area at LSHT mile 75	N 30°32.759' W 95°07.833'

SUPPLIES AND ACCOMMODATIONS

From Evergreen, at LSHT mile 65.0, it is approximately 14.5 miles to New Waverly (population: 950) east on Highway 150. New Waverly does not offer any overnight lodging, but does have several combination gas

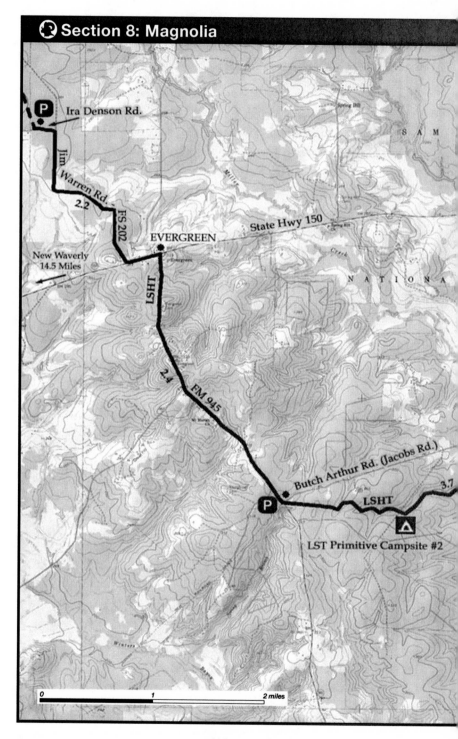

Ira Denson Rd.

Jim Warren Rd.

2.2

FS 202

EVERGREEN

State Hwy 150

New Waverly
14.5 Miles

LSHT

2.4

FM 945

Butch Arthur Rd. (Jacobs Rd.)

3.7

LSHT

LST Primitive Campsite #2

SAM

NATIONA

0   1   2 miles

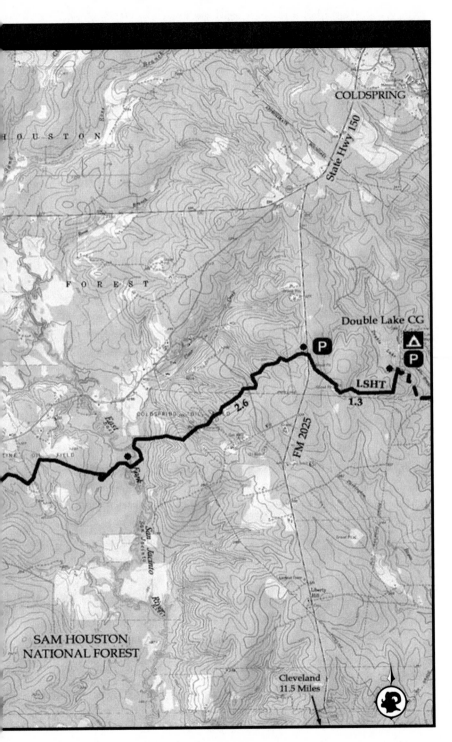

COLDSPRING

State Hwy 150

H O U S T O N

F O R E S T

Double Lake CG

P

LSHT

2.6

1.3

FM 2025

San Jacinto River

SAM HOUSTON
NATIONAL FOREST

Cleveland
11.5 Miles

station and convenience stores, restaurants, and a grocery store. In the other direction, from Evergreen, it is 9 miles to Coldspring (population: 691) east on Highway 150. Coldspring does not offer any overnight lodging, but does offer a local diner, barbeque restaurant, post office, dollar store, gas stations, and a grocery store. The full-service town of Shepherd (population: 2,262) along U.S. Highway 59 is 11 miles southeast of Coldspring and offers several motels.

Double Lake Recreation Area offers campsites ($16 per night) equipped with picnic tables and campfire rings or a cooking grill. Hot showers, bathrooms with running water, and potable water taps are located throughout the campground, as are vending machines and pay phones. In the warmer months on weekends, a concession stand may be set up in the park.

WATER

Along the 4.6-mile road walk at the western end of Section 8, there is no water available, even though you pass through the town of Evergreen. However, once you are hiking in the woods, the Magnolia Section provides regular water sources. Many of the smaller streams dry up in warmer months, but the East Fork of the San Jacinto River is reliable in any season (though the water here can be extremely silt-laden). At the eastern end of Section 8, potable water is available just 0.2 mile off the LSHT in the Double Lake Recreation Area (or can be taken from the lake itself adjacent to the trail at mile 75.0).

TRAIL DESCRIPTION

From LSHT Trailhead Parking Lot #9, begin this section's 4.6-mile road walk by turning left onto dirt Ira

Denson Road from where the trail exits the woods into the parking lot. (Remember that if you are westbound, you need to reverse all directions, left and right, in these trail descriptions.) Walk beneath the power lines 0.2 mile to the intersection with dirt FS 202. Turn right onto FS 202 and cross under the power lines again. After 0.5 mile, at LSHT mile 63.5, you'll notice the first farmland along the road. Houses begin to appear soon after.

Reach the intersection of FS 202 (named John Warren Road) and Highway 150 after 2.7 miles on FS 202, at LSHT mile 64.7. Turn left onto Highway 150, walk 0.3 mile past the first road that intersects the highway on the left and a red brick building on the right. Continue until you reach the intersection of Highway 150 and FM 945 at a flashing stoplight at LSHT mile 65.0. This is downtown Evergreen, which offers no services to the road-weary hiker (the larger town of Coldspring is about 8 miles east on Highway 150).

Turn right onto FM 945 at this intersection. MILE MARKERS 63, 64, 65, 66, and 67 are passed on this road walk, although they are most likely not marked along the roads. Pass a cemetery on the left at mile 65.5 and top a rise at mile 66.0. You pass another cemetery, some houses, and a pretty pond before reaching LSHT mile 67.4 and the intersection of FM 945 with Butch Arther Road (also known as Jacobs Road). LSHT Trailhead Parking Lot #10 offers shady parking and a trailhead bulletin board near where the trail heads back into the woods at long last. From this point to the eastern terminus, the LSHT has National Recreation Trail status. (The road walk on FM 945 measured at a total of 2.7 miles by three different measuring tools, indicating that this LSHT segment is short by 0.3 mile. You should actually be at LSHT mile 67.7, not 67.4, once you reach Parking Lot #10. However, to stay consistent with the trail mile markers, this guide ignores those extra 0.3 mile that, unfortunately, your feet cannot.)

Now back in the woods, cross a seasonal drainage at mile 67.9 and soon after pass **MILE MARKER 68**. Very thick undergrowth prevents camping in a flat area of mature pines. In the springtime, watch for the slender wakerobin, also known as the Sabine River wakerobin (*Trillium gracile*), growing near steams; trilliums are three-petaled wildflowers only rarely spotted in the Sam Houston National Forest. Cross a large seasonal drainage on a hiker bridge at mile 68.2 and soon discover a woodland of mature Southern magnolia trees that are this section's namesake. Cross back over the drainage, which may have a bit of water in it during wet seasons. Reach the LSHT Primitive Campsite #2 **Campsite** ▲ at mile 68.6; ▲ this backcountry site lies just off the LSHT to the right along an access trail. Several cleared tent sites and a fire ring sit in a large open area, making a convenient site for an overnight stay. You'll need to pack in water, however.

With magnolias shading overhead in every season and honeysuckle blooming profusely in the spring, pass **MILE MARKER 69** in a tree to the right of the trail. Just after, at mile 69.1, pass a fence corner on the left. As you notice a larger creek that usually has some water in it, you will also notice a parcel of private land off to the left. It is best not to camp in this area. Several large oil and gas fields lie just north of the national forest. At mile 69.3, pass another fence corner and cross over the creek, which you will parallel and cross several times ahead. As an interesting note, you are walking at an elevation of 262 feet above sea level.

At mile 69.8, reach a junction with an ATV track where you can spot a picturesque horse farm through the trees to the right. The trail here is often misused by equestrians who are not supposed to be riding on the LSHT. Pass the dirt road that leads up the drive of the horse farm and pass **MILE MARKER 70**. The creek you have been crossing multiple times appears again, spanned now by a crooked bridge; this creek drains into the East Fork of the San Jacinto River. Just after you cross the bridge, a sign directs you to make a sharp right-hand turn. The trail follows an old road bed, passing a sad wetland on private property that appears to have been clearcut. Nevertheless, watch for pileated woodpeckers and barred owls, which I have spotted near here. The LSHT continues to be wide and easy to walk. Large, striking magnolias appear regularly. Wherever they grow, Southern magnolias indicate a subtropical climate.

Reach a hiker gate at mile 70.6. An old road heads off to the left, but you remain on the LSHT straight

Flooding destroyed the LSHT footbridge over the East Fork of the San Jacinto River in 2005. It has yet to be repaired as of fall 2009.

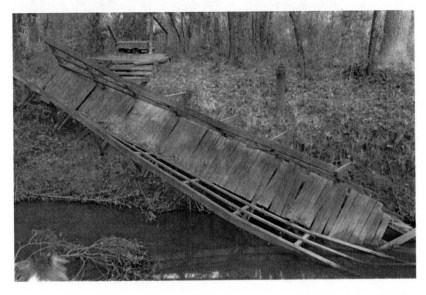

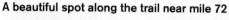

A beautiful spot along the trail near mile 72

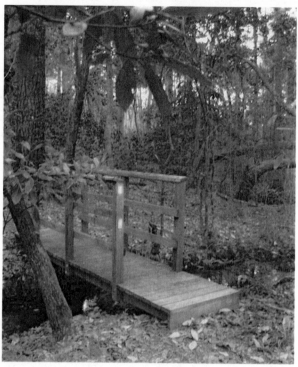

ahead. Some ATV misuse of the trail may be evident. An extremely varied forest emerges at **MILE MARKER 71**; wetlands mix with hardwoods, pines, and palmettos. Intersect an orange-striped trail soon after. Follow the LSHT trail markers straight ahead to the banks of the East Fork of the San Jacinto River.

When I hiked the trail, the hiker bridge had been washed out by high water. Fording the river required a thigh-deep wade through coffee-colored waters and a slippery ascent up the far bank. Hopefully, you will find the hiker bridge intact. Don't filter your drinking water here; just ahead at mile 71.3 is a tributary of the river that normally runs with deep, clear water. This tributary is also bridged, as is the next shallow clear stream at mile 71.7. This area supports a variety of hardwood trees and vines that give it the otherworldly appearance of an ancient jungle. Begin climbing out of the river's bottom-lands, paralleling an old barbed wire fence on the left.

MILE MARKER 72 is reached in drier pine uplands just before a pipeline right-of-way and jeep track. Head downhill now into an interesting rolling area filled with sweetbay, holly, and magnolia. As you reach the bottom of the draw, find one of the jewels of the LSHT, a beauti-ful hiker bridge spanning a clear creek with a tiny water-fall. At this spot, from August to October, you may find an uncommon, often overlooked, saprophytic (feeds off of dead and decaying plant material) in the form of a delicate flowering annual called the nodding nixie. This is also a good place to look for snakes and frogs.

At mile 72.3, you may notice a flat spot left of the trail that would make a nice campsite cushioned by pine needles. ▲ Cross a good gravel road and utili- **▲ Campsite** ties right-of-way at mile 72.4. Cross an old logging road at mile 72.6; a clearing is visible to the right. At mile 72.8, reach an old roadbed and make a sharp right to follow the road. Pass through a metal gate at mile 72.9 and over a wide logging road. Just past MILE MARKER 73, make a sharp turn to the right that can be very easy to overlook. A nice long hiker bridge spans a seasonal gully at mile 73.1. The forest's character has changed to include a wider variety of trees since you crossed the East Fork of the San Jacinto River.

Reach FM 2025 at mile 73.7 and continue straight across this paved road. LSHT Trailhead Park-ing Lot #11 is located here on the east side of FM 2025. Cross under utility lines (there are some open areas here that could serve as campsites, ▲ although they **▲ Campsite** are very close to the road and most likely contain some litter) and through several hiker gates. Reach **MILE MARKER 74** where thick young undergrowth prevents any further thoughts of camping until you reach an

Campsite ▲ open area at mile 74.8. ▲ However, you are now very near the developed campgrounds of Double Lake Recreation Area. The trail soon turns into a semipaved surface as it reaches the outskirts of the park's nature trail system. Cross an old road at mile 74.9 and continue straight ahead. At LSHT **MILE MARKER 75**, break out of the woods by a large LSHT sign. You'll see spring-fed Double Lake directly ahead. To reach the park's facilities, leave the LSHT here, turn left, and walk along the edge of the lake for a few minutes.

Double Lake Recreation Area offers campsites ($16 per night), hot showers, bathrooms with running water, potable water taps, pay phones, and vending machines. Canoes and paddleboats can be rented at the *seasonal* concession stand that may also sell snacks and groceries. The LSHT comes out at the corner of one of the lakes, then turns immediately back into the woods, and does not continue to Double Lake Recreation Area's facilities. To enter the developed campground, follow the shoreline of the lake toward the buildings visible from the trail. To continue eastbound on the trail: At the large LSHT sign at mile 75 while facing the lake, make a hard right turn back into the woods and enter Section 9. *Do not continue straight ahead along the top of the lake's dam.*

SECTION 8 MILEAGE

MILES W→E	TRAIL POINT	MILES E→W	NOTES
62.8	LSHT Big Woods Trailhead Parking Lot #9; follow LSHT left onto dirt Ira Denson Road	33.3	▬ 🅿
63.0	MILE MARKER 63; intersection of Ira Denson Rd. and FS 202	33.1	▬
64.0	MILE MARKER 64	32.1	
64.7	Intersection of FS 202 (John Warren Rd.) and Hwy. 150; follow LSHT left on Hwy. 150	31.4	▬
65.0	MILE MARKER 65; intersection of Hwy. 150 and FM 945 in Evergreen; follow LSHT right on FM 945	31.1	▬
65.5	Cemetery on left along FM 945	30.6	
66.0	MILE MARKER 66	30.1	
67.0	MILE MARKER 67	29.1	
67.4	Intersection of FM 945 and Butch Arther Rd. (Jacobs Rd.); LSHT Trailhead Parking Lot #10	28.7	▬ 🅿
67.9	Seasonal drainage	28.2	
68.0	MILE MARKER 68	28.1	
68.2	Hiker bridge over large seasonal drainage (low flow; good water)	27.9	🚰 *
68.4	Seasonal drainage	27.7	
68.6	LSHT Primitive Campsite #2 to right of trail	27.5	▲
69.0	MILE MARKER 69	27.1	
69.1	Fence corner	27.0	
69.2	Creek (low flow; good water)	26.9	🚰 *
69.3	Fence corner	26.8	
69.4	Creek (low flow; good water)	26.7	🚰 *
69.8	ATV track; horse farm	26.3	
69.9	Dirt road	26.2	
70.0	MILE MARKER 70	26.1	
70.1	Hiker bridge over drainage (low flow; good water)	26.0	🚰 *
70.6	Hiker gate; stay straight	25.5	
71.0	MILE MARKER 71; intersect orange-striped trail; follow LSHT straight	25.1	
71.1	Bridge over East Fork San Jacinto River	25.0	🚰
71.3	Hiker bridge over creek (deep, clear water)	24.8	🚰
71.7	Hiker bridge over stream (shallow, clear water)	24.4	🚰 *

SECTION 8 MILEAGE

MILES W→E	TRAIL POINT	MILES E→W	NOTES
72.0	**MILE MARKER 72;** pipeline right-of-way; gravel jeep track	24.1	
72.2	Hiker bridge over creek (shallow, clear water)	23.9	🚰 *
72.3	Potential campsite on left	23.8	▲
72.4	Gravel road; utilities right-of-way	23.7	
72.6	Old logging road; clearing to the right	23.5	
72.8	Old roadbed; make sharp right turn and follow old road	23.3	
72.9	Metal gate; logging road	23.2	
73.0	**MILE MARKER 73**	23.1	
73.1	Sharp right turn; hiker bridge over seasonal drainage	23.0	
73.7	FM 2025; LSHT Trailhead Parking Lot #11	22.4	➖ 🅿
73.8	Potential camping (close to road); utility lines	22.3	▲
73.9	Two hiker gates	22.2	
74.0	**MILE MARKER 74**	22.1	
74.8	Open area; reach gravel nature trail on top of old railroad bed; potential camping	21.3	▲
74.9	Old road	21.2	
75.0	Double Lake Recreation Area; **MILE MARKER 75**	21.1	➖ 🚰 🅿 🏕

* Water here is seasonal and dependent on weather conditions.

MILEAGE CHART KEY

🚰	Water source	▲	Undeveloped campsite or potential camping area
🏕	Developed campground		
🅿	Parking area/trailhead	➖	Major roads (jeep tracks and logging roads are not indicated)

Double Lake Recreation Area to
Farm to Market 2666

OVERVIEW

Many find the Big Creek Section of the LSHT *to be the* highlight of the entire trail. The most diverse along the 96-mile LSHT, the beautiful forests are filled with nearly every species of tree that can be found in the bottomland and upland forests of East Texas. Double Lake is spring fed, making it unusually clear and cool for a small lake in this region. The lake feeds one of the major tributaries of Big Creek, which grows increasingly larger and more scenic as it runs toward the 1,420-acre Big Creek Scenic Area. In fact, numerous perennial streams and creeks feed into this protected area, resulting in a lush pine–hardwood forest filled with a variety of flora and fauna. Bird-watchers are particularly enamored with the Big Creek Section.

The LSHT itself remains well marked, including a newly rerouted section that moves the trail away from the erosion-prone banks of upper Big Creek. The hike covers rolling ground up along the banks of the creek and down into its bottomlands. There are a few muddy areas, but several are conveniently traversed by boardwalks. Every creek in this section is crossed by a hiker bridge, so there is no worry about having to ford them in rainy weather.

Camping is prohibited within the boundaries of the Big Creek Scenic Area. To reduce impact in this beautiful section, plan to camp in either the developed Double Lake Recreation Area at mile 75 (fee required) or the semideveloped backcountry site (no fee) simply named LSHT Primitive Campsite #1 at mile 75.7. Four small loop trails connect to the LSHT within the

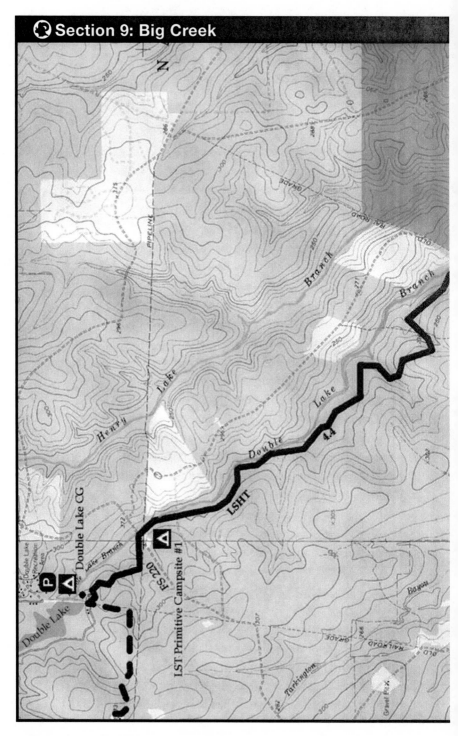

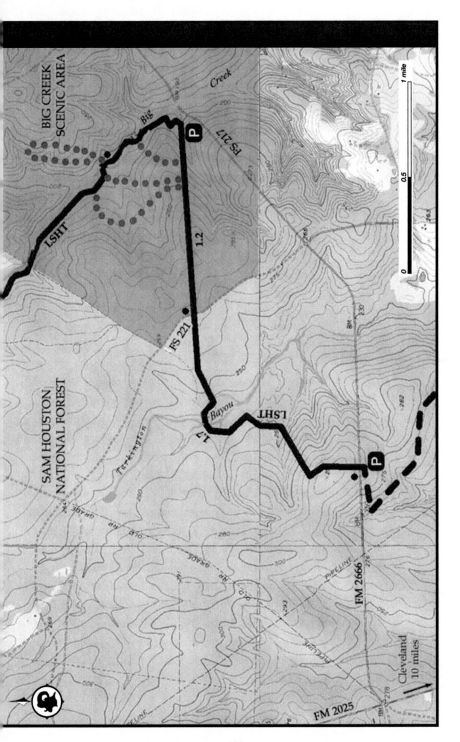

BIG CREEK SCENIC AREA

SAM HOUSTON NATIONAL FOREST

LSHT

LSHT

Big

Creek

Bayou

Turkington

FS 217

FS 221

1.2

1.7

LSHT

FM 2666

FM 2025

Cleveland
10 miles

PIPELINE

RR GRADE

OLD RR GRADE

0   0.5   1 mile

boundaries of the Big Creek Scenic Area, making this an excellent section for dayhiking.

TRAIL ACCESS AND PARKING

To reach Double Lake Recreation Area, take Highway 150 from Evergreen 5.7 miles east to Farm to Market (FM) 2025 (or 25 miles east from New Waverly). Turn right (south) onto FM 2025 for 0.4 mile and turn left onto Double Lake Park Road. Ask camp hosts about parking a car within the recreation area; there is a $6 fee per day to park here. Potable tap water is available at the campground.

To reach the Big Creek Scenic Area and LSHT Trailhead Parking Lot #12 (near LSHT mile 79.9) from the town of Shepherd along U.S. Highway 59, head west on Highway 150 for about 5 miles. Forest Service (FS) Road 217 is a small paved road that comes in from the left. Turn left (southeast) on FS 217 and follow it for 1.8 miles. The gravel LSHT Trailhead Parking Lot #12 will be on the right. A short side trail leads to the LSHT from the parking lot. Nonpotable water can be found in Big Creek just a short walk westbound on the LSHT.

To reach the eastern end of Section 9 (at LSHT mile 82.3) at the LSHT Trailhead Parking Lot #13 along Farm to Market (FM) 2666, from the town of Shepherd along U.S. Highway 59 head west on Highway 150 for about 1.5 miles. FM 2666 meets Highway 150 on the left. Turn left onto FM 2666 and follow it for 6.5 miles. LSHT Trailhead Parking Lot #13 is signed and visible on the right side of FM 2666. There is ample parking, a trash can, and bulletin board, but no drinking water.

SECTION 9 GPS Waypoints	
Double Lake Recreation Area at LSHT mile 75	N 30°32.759' W 95°07.833'
Primitive Campsite #1 at LSHT mile 75.7	N 30°32.466' W 95°07.419'
LSHT Trailhead Parking Lot #12 at Big Creek Scenic Area	N 30°30.333' W 95°05.314'
LSHT Tarkington Trailhead Parking Lot #13 on FM 2666	N 30°29.558' W 95°07.111'

SUPPLIES AND ACCOMMODATIONS

Double Lake Recreation Area offers campsites ($16 per night) equipped with picnic tables, campfire rings, and cooking grills. Hot showers, bathrooms with running water, and potable water taps are located throughout the campground, as are vending machines and pay phones. In the warmer months on weekends, a concession stand may be set up in the park. These facilities are a few minutes' walk from the LSHT. From mile 75 and the large LSHT sign by the southwest corner of the lake, turn left and head into the campground, which is visible from this spot (the LSHT continues to the right).

The town of Coldspring is about 4 miles from Double Lake, northeast on Highway 150. Coldspring (population: 691) does not offer any overnight lodging, but does offer a local diner, barbeque restaurant, post office, dollar store, gas stations, and a large grocery store. The larger, full-service town of Shepherd (population: 2,262) along U.S. Highway 59 is 11 miles southeast of Coldspring and offers several motels.

Shepherd can also be accessed from the eastern, or southern, end of Section 9. From FM 2666 and LSHT Trailhead Parking Lot #13, follow FM 2666 about 6.5 miles east. Turn right (east) on Highway 150 and follow it 1.5 miles into Shepherd. From LSHT Trailhead Parking Lot #12 in the Big Creek Scenic Area, follow FS 217 northeast a few miles to intersect Highway 150. Shepherd is about 5 miles to the east.

The spring-fed waters of Double Lake at LSHT mile 75

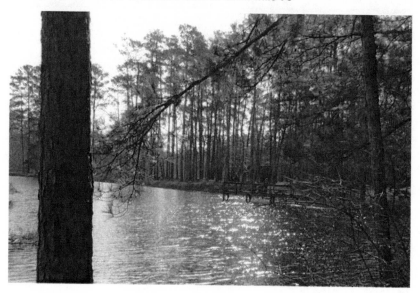

WATER

The Big Creek Section is blessed with abundant water. At the shoreline of spring-fed Double Lake, it is short walk off-trail to its developed recreation facilities (where potable tap water is available) at the western end of this LSHT section at mile 75. As the hiker heads into the middle region of this section, the trail parallels Double Lake Branch and, later, Big Creek. These spring-fed creeks flow year-round with clear water that is easily the most appealing of any groundwater along the entire LSHT. Only toward the eastern end of Section 9, from mile 79.8 to mile 82.3, is water scarce.

TRAIL DESCRIPTION

The LSHT intersects Double Lake on the shoreline at the far southwest corner of the lake by a large LSHT sign at mile 75.0. The LSHT skirts, but does not enter Double Lake Recreation Area's facilities. The trail continues eastbound from the large LSHT sign at mile 75; while facing the lake at the sign, make a hard right turn back into the woods to enter Section 9. Do not continue straight ahead on the trail across the lake's dam. (Remember that if you are westbound, you need to reverse all directions, left and right, in these trail descriptions.)

You soon cross a utilities right-of-way and intersect one of the recreation area's mountain biking trails. At mile 75.3, meet up with a short boardwalk over a wet section. Cross an old fence line and reach another short boardwalk. Notice a transition into picturesque moist woodland dominated by evergreen shrubs, vines, and ferns. Cross gravel Forest Service (FS) Road 220 and proceed through a hiker gate across the road and over a large creek that drains Double Lake at mile 75.6. This is a main tributary of Big Creek named Double Lake Branch, which you follow for the next 4 miles (though mostly at a distance). Cross a tiny bridge over a seasonal drainage and reach LSHT Primitive Campsite #1 at mile 75.7, ▲ **▲ Campsite** which has four tent pads. Water is available back at the road in the creek that drains the lake.

Just after this signed turnoff, you may notice signs indicating that the LSHT has been rerouted due to erosion along the banks of the creek. Due to this reroute, the LSHT has grown in length by 0.3 mile. Again, this guide ignores this extra 0.3 mile to maintain consistency with the existing LSHT mile markers.

Hence, the LSHT turns slightly uphill on new tread into the higher woodland of loblolly pine.

MILE MARKER 76 should appear soon, but it is probably not marked on this new trail tread. Damage to large trees, especially down by the creek, is probably due to a past storm, but there are places to make camp through-

Campsite ▲ out this area. ▲ Reach the creek's banks again at mile 76.4. It may be shallow, but is usually flowing and clear. Cross a small hiker bridge over a deep seasonal drainage and ignore a split in the trail that soon joins together again. Cross over a long, narrow bridge at mile 76.6, merging with another trail (that may be the original LSHT tread) and staying to the right.

If you have a sharp eye for trees, you may notice a pure stand of swamp chestnut oaks (*Quercus michauxii*). Mature leaves can be up to 11 inches long (though are typically between 4 and 8 inches in length), broad and oval with rounded, simple teeth. The large acorns of this bottomland-dwelling oak taste extra sweet to livestock, giving the swamp chestnut oak its nickname of "cow oak." As you proceed along the banks of Double Lake Branch, you pass Southern magnolias, American hollies, red oaks, beeches, sycamores, and hickories—to name only a few of the tree species that thrive here.

Pass a set of bridges just before **MILE MARKER 77** (actually, this is an orange post that reads only 7). Cross a small drainage and proceed along the side of the hill. Cross the creek again at 77.6 where the water tends to stagnate at times. **MILE MARKER 78** may not be in place yet either, but should be located at the apex of a small climb. At mile 78.6, cross an old railroad trestle, following signs through a new hiker gate.

You are now entering the Big Creek Scenic Area where no camping or hunting is allowed (you may begin to look for camping after LSHT mile 80.6). The trail can be very muddy through here, but hiker bridges

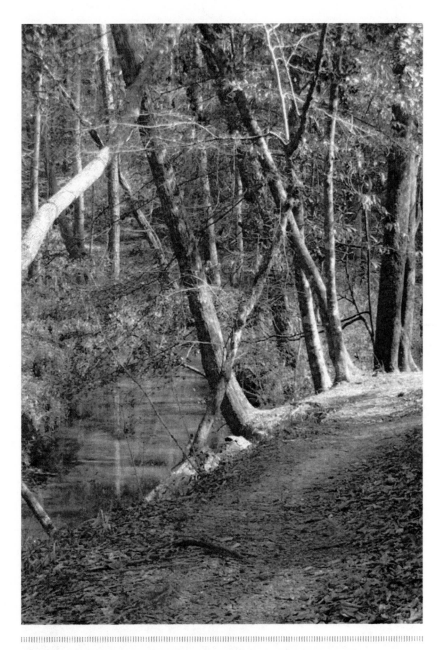

The LSHT parallels scenic Double Lake Branch just upstream of its confluence with Henry Lake Branch.

and boardwalks cover the worst areas. **MILE MARKER 79** should be located just after one bridge near where a huge sycamore carved with thoughtless graffiti grows to the right of the trail. Mosquitoes frequent this area, even in cooler months.

Reach the junction of Double Lake Branch with Big Creek's other main tributary, Henry Lake Branch. A little waterfall graces this spot. A sign tells you that you've come 4 miles since Double Lake, which is fairly accurate. Cross a big bridge and intersect an orange-blazed trail (the Big Creek Trail) that heads off to the right. Follow the LSHT left. Cross a swampy spot that is bridged and reach LSHT **MILE MARKER 79** (this is the old mile marker, which is now located 0.3 mile beyond where it should be on the reroute).

Next, you'll see a signed junction of the White Oak Trail, a green-blazed trail that heads off to the

A view of Big Creek from the LSHT

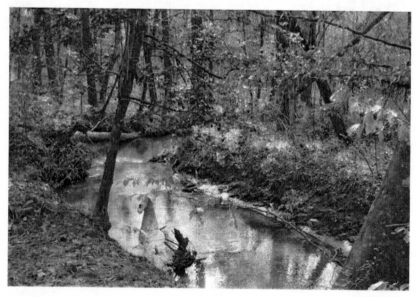

right. Stay straight on the LSHT and immediately cross a bridge over Big Creek's clear waters. Pass a tiny bridge and the permanently closed Magnolia Trail (once blue-blazed) on the left. Follow the LSHT to the right and through a muddy area. A long hiker bridge slopes slightly, but is passable at mile 79.5. Continue to parallel Big Creek, which is to the right. With beech trees leaning over its banks and clear, deep waters, spring-fed Big Creek is especially scenic.

Cross another long bridge and reach a junction with the yellow-striped Pine Trail, which heads off to the right. Follow the LSHT to the left. Cross another bridge and make a sharp right turn where you should see a large sign with a map of the Big Creek Scenic Area etched upon it at LSHT mile 79.9. A trail heads off to the left and to LSHT Big Creek Scenic Area Trailhead Parking Lot #12 where there is a bench, information board, and trash can.

Alternate Big Creek Scenic Area Loop Trails:
· PINE LOOP, YELLOW-BLAZED, 0.14 MILE
· WHITE OAK LOOP, GREEN-BLAZED, 0.45 MILE
· BIG CREEK LOOP, ORANGE-BLAZED, 0.63 MILE
· NOW CLOSED: MAGNOLIA LOOP, BLUE-STRIPED, 0.61 MILE

Here the trail begins its southwestern arc; east-bound hikers may notice that they are heading due west for a few miles before turning south. As you continue down the LSHT, you may notice a yellow-blazed trail (the other end of the Pine Trail) heading off to the right, followed by a couple of trailside benches and the orange-striped Big Creek Trail off to the right (the White Oak Trail also joins the LSHT again at this point). Soon, reach **MILE MARKER 80**, which is marked 5. If you haven't already noticed, you are walking on top of an old road or railroad bed, which may have served the logging industry in the past. Cross a hiker gate at mile 80.6 and proceed straight across gravel road Forest Service (FS) Road 221, leaving the scenic area. Immediately, the diverse ecosystem of the Big Creek area is replaced by a homogenous young pine plantation.

Cross a small seasonal drainage and pass **MILE MARKER 81**. At mile 81.2, cross an unidentified trail and follow the LSHT left. Waterless camping ▲ could be made in an open spot here. Cross several more seasonal drainages, including the ephemeral channel of Tarkington Bayou, where the trail may be muddy in wet seasons. Continue to walk in and out of hardwood bottomland and young pine forests. At mile 81.9, there is another small waterless campsite ▲ just before you enter a mature forest of white ash, black hickory, and white oak. Reach **MILE MARKER 82** and continue onward to the LSHT Tarkington Trailhead Parking Lot #13 along FM 2666 at LSHT mile 82.3.

Campsite ▲ (first)
Campsite ▲ (second)

SECTION 9 MILEAGE

MILES W→E	TRAIL POINT	MILES E→W	NOTES
75.0	Double Lake Recreation Area; **MILE MARKER 75**	21.1	🚻 🚰 P
75.1	Utilities right-of-way; intersect mountain biking trail	21.0	
75.6	Gravel FS 220; hiker gate; Big Creek tributary on left	20.5	🚻 🚰
75.7	Hiker bridge over seasonal drainage; LSHT Primitive Campsite #1; begin marked trail reroute on higher ground above creek	20.4	▲
76.0	Small bridge over deep drainage; potential camping; creek on left (good water; low flow); **MILE MARKER 76***	20.1	🚰 ▲
76.5	Small bridge over deep drainage	19.6	
76.6	Long bridge over creek; follow LSHT right	19.5	
76.9	Two bridges over small creeks (low flow; good water)	19.2	🚰
77.0	**MILE MARKER 77***	19.1	
77.6	Cross swampy creek (stagnant water)	18.5	

SECTION 9 MILEAGE

MILES W→E	TRAIL POINT	MILES E→W	NOTES
78.0	**MILE MARKER 78***	18.1	
78.6	Cross old railroad bed; veer left to follow LSHT through hiker gate	17.5	
79.0	**MILE MARKER 79***	17.1	
79.2	Intersect orange-blazed Big Creek Trail; follow LSHT left	16.9	
79.3	**ORIGINAL MILE MARKER 79;** intersect green-blazed White Oak Trail; follow LSHT left	16.8	⚱
79.4	Bridge over Big Creek; intersect permanently closed, blue-blazed Magnolia Loop Trail; follow LSHT right	16.7	⚱
79.7	Long bridge over Big Creek; intersect yellow-blazed Pine Trail; follow LSHT left	16.4	⚱
79.8	Hiker bridge; intersect trail heading down to left; follow LSHT's sharp right turn	16.3	
79.9	Big Creek Scenic Area sign; short side trail to left leads to LSHT Trailhead Parking Lot #12; intersect yellow-blazed Pine Trail and orange-blazed Big Creek Trail on right; follow LSHT straight ahead on old railroad bed	16.2	🅿
80.0	**MILE MARKER 80** (this "mile" is 1.3 miles long due to reroute)	16.1	
80.6	Hiker gate; gravel FS 221	15.5	▭
81.0	Small seasonal drainage; **MILE MARKER 81**	15.1	
81.2	Intersect unidentified trail; follow LSHT left; potential campsite; seasonal drainage	14.9	▲
82.0	**MILE MARKER 82**	14.1	
82.3	LSHT Tarkington Trailhead Parking Lot #13; FM 2666	13.8	▭ 🅿

* LSHT mile markers are not yet in place on rerouted trail.

MILEAGE CHART KEY

⚱ Water source	▲ Undeveloped campsite or potential camping area
🚐 Developed campground	
🅿 Parking area/trailhead	▭ Major roads (jeep tracks and logging roads are not indicated)

Farm to Market 2666 to Farm to Market 1725

OVERVIEW

The term bayou *probably originated from* the Choctaw word for "small stream," and was first used by the French in the Louisiana territory to denote a slow-moving creek located in a relatively flat, low area. Section 10 provides the hiker with the opportunity for an up-close encounter with several East Texas bayous and their rich ecosystems. Popular culture has often cast bayous in the role of spooky, mysterious places where overhung moss darkens junglelike forests.

Come out and hike the Bayou Section of the LSHT to see for yourself—you may find, as you stroll along the banks of Tarkington Bayou or cross the larger Winters Bayou, that bayous and their surrounding lands are unique. Indeed, many forest creatures depend on their slow-moving waters for homes. Trees of all types live in these bottomlands; plants uncommon in other sections of the LSHT—leafy vines, ferns, and palms—are abundant here.

The trail in Section 10 traverses the lowest elevation along the entire LSHT, around 160 feet above sea level, so not only is this area blessed with many creeks and drainages, but it also tends to flood during wet seasons. In fact, during heavy rains, expect to be wading in ankle-deep water in several places. The larger streams are all bridged, two with dependable steel-foot bridges. The trail is easy to follow in all but a couple of spots mentioned below. However, the wonders of the Bayou Section are probably best discovered in drier seasons—or, in wet periods, left to those with proper footwear and the adventurous spirit necessary for exploring a primeval landscape of beautiful lowlands.

TRAIL ACCESS AND PARKING

To reach the western, or northern end of Section 10 (at LSHT mile 82.3) at the LSHT Trailhead Parking Lot #13 along Farm to Market (FM) 2666, from the town of Shepherd along U.S. Highway 59, head west on Highway 150 for about 1.5 miles. FM 2666 meets Highway 150 on the left. Turn left onto FM 2666 and follow it for 6.5 miles. LSHT Trailhead Parking Lot #13 is signed and visible on the right side of FM 2666. There is ample parking, a trash can, and bulletin board, but no drinking water.

To reach LSHT Trailhead Parking Lot #14 on Farm to Market (FM) 2025 from Cleveland, take FM 2025 approximately 7 miles from Cleveland. The parking lot is on the right side of the road.

To reach the LSHT crossing of Highway 945 (at LSHT mile 93.0) from Cleveland along U.S. Highway 59, follow FM 2025 north for 6.5 miles to the junction with Highway 945. There is a gas station on the left at this intersection. Turn onto Highway 945 and go 1.4 miles, watching for LSHT signs pointing out the location of the trail as it crosses the road. There is not a parking lot or trailhead here.

To reach the eastern, or southern, end and terminus of the LSHT (at LSHT mile 96.1) along Farm to Market (FM) 1725 from Cleveland, follow Highway 105 for 1 mile from U.S. Highway 59. Turn right (northwest) on FM 1725 and go 5.2 miles to reach LSHT Trailhead Parking Lot #15, which is on the right side of the road just before a white church building (Montague Church). There is a bulletin board, ample

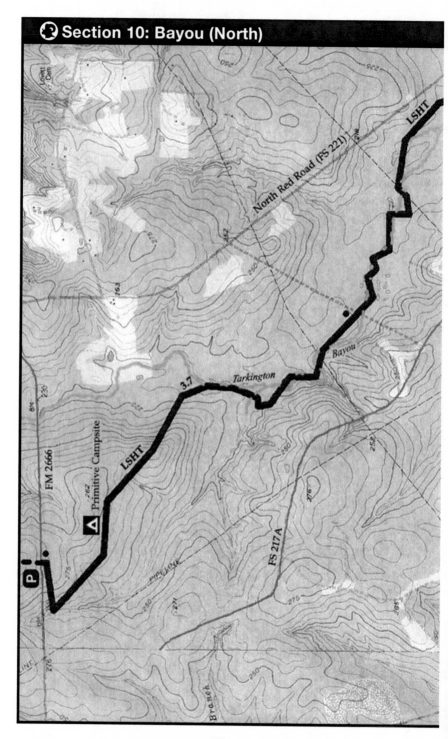

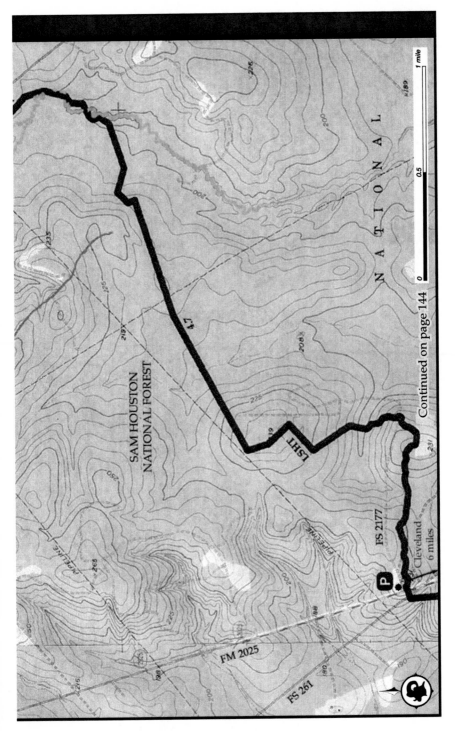

SAM HOUSTON
NATIONAL FOREST

NATIONAL

LSHT

FS 2177

Cleveland
6 miles

FM 2025

FS 261

parent

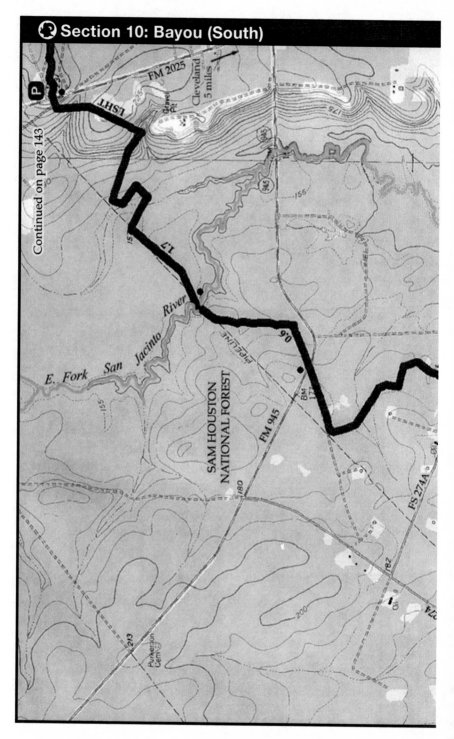

Continued on page 143

FM 2025

Cleveland
5 miles

LSHT

Gravel
Pit

945

155

15

17

90

E. Fork San Jacinto River

PIPELINE

SAM HOUSTON
NATIONAL FOREST

FM 945

BM

180

FS 274A

182

200

203

Parkerson
Cem.

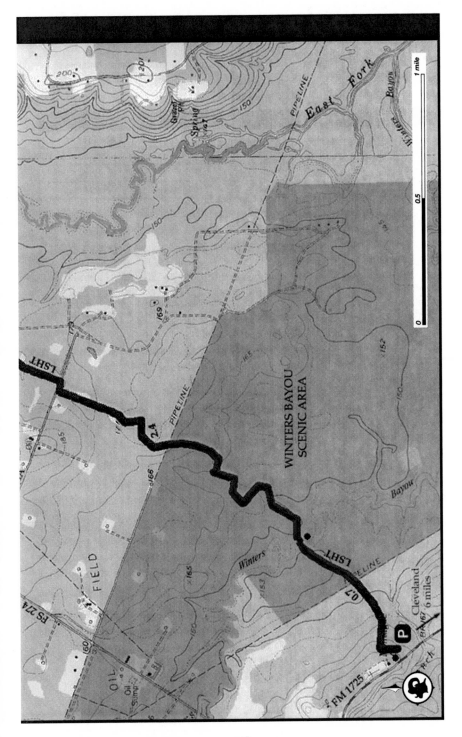

WINTERS BAYOU SCENIC AREA

East Fork

Winters Bayou

Spring

FIELD

OIL

Winters
Bayou

LHST

LHST

PIPELINE

PIPELINE

FS 274

FM 1725

Cleveland
6 miles

0   0.5   1 mile

parking, and a trash can, but no drinking water at this parking area.

SECTION 10 GPS Waypoints	
LSHT Trailhead Parking Lot #13 on FM 2666	N 30°29.558' W 95°07.111'
LSHT Trailhead Parking Lot #14 on FM 2025	N 30°26.312' W 95°07.268'
Intersection with Highway 945 at LSHT mile 93	N 30°25.381' W 95°08.328'
LSHT Trailhead Parking Lot #15 on FM 1725	N 30°23.593' W 95°09.484'

SUPPLIES AND ACCOMMODATIONS

The full-service town of Shepherd (population: 2,262) is about 8 miles from the eastern end of Section 9 and offers motels, restaurants, a post office, and many other businesses. From FM 2666 and LSHT Trailhead Parking Lot #13, follow FM 2666 about 6.5 miles east. Turn right (east) on Highway 150 and follow it 1.5 miles into Shepherd.

The large, full-service town of Cleveland (population: 8,046) is approximately 6 miles southeast of LSHT Trailhead Parking Lot #14 at the junction of FM 2025 and U.S. Highway 59. Cleveland can also be reached easily from the LSHT crossing of Highway 945 (LSHT mile 93) by heading east on Highway 945 for 1.4 miles and turning south on FM 2025 for 6.5 miles. From the eastern terminus of the LSHT at mile 96.1 and LSHT Trailhead Parking Lot #15, you can reach Cleveland by taking FM 1725 southeast for 5.2 miles and turning east on Highway 105 for 1 mile. When you reach U.S. Highway 59, turn north for a mile or so to reach the town center. Cleveland offers several motels and a good selection of stores and restaurants.

WATER

Section 10 has more groundwater than any other LSHT section and has regularly spaced water sources. Tarkington Bayou, which the LSHT follows for several miles, is intermittent and cannot be relied upon in dry seasons. The large perennial creek, Winters Bayou, is always reliable, although its waters tend to be muddy and its banks steep and slippery. Several smaller tributaries and streams feed into these bottomlands, many of which flow clear and strong most of the year though they cannot be relied upon in very dry seasons.

TRAIL DESCRIPTION

From the LSHT Tarkington Trailhead Parking Lot #13 along FM 2666 at LSHT mile 82.3, cross the highway and continue to parallel it on trail for a few minutes

The East Fork of the San Jacinto River in the Bayou Section

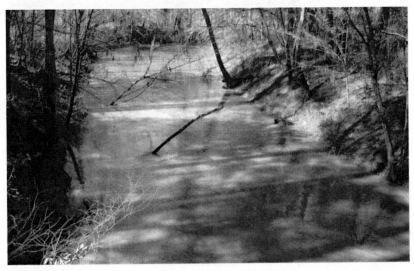

A hiker at the steel hiker bridge over the East Fork of the San Jacinto River

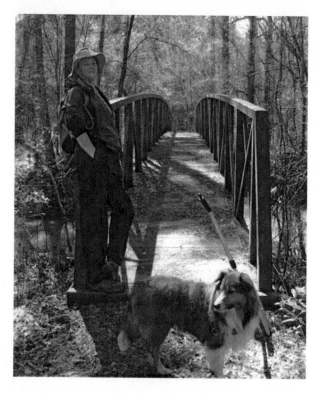

in a pine plantation. Reach a hiker gate at mile 82.6. The rolling land you've experienced since crossing the East Fork of the San Jacinto River back in Section 8 (if you're thru-hiking) is now gone; here you are walking through long stretches of pure pine forests on flat ground. Longleaf pines, rare along the LSHT, grow in this area. The longleaf pine is highly resistant to fire and, prior to suppression of wildfire by European settlers, was the dominant pine in the southern U.S. It remains in only 5 percent of its former range.

Pass **MILE MARKER 83** among brushy undergrowth. At mile 83.2, you may notice a corner benchmark and bearing tree (identified by the yellow sign affixed to its trunk, a bearing tree serves as an official survey marker) near an ATV or horse trail. Reach a signed primitive campsite to the left of the trail (no water is available at this campsite). ▲ Cross a seasonal drainage on a new hiker bridge at mile 83.4 and another without a bridge at mile 83.7. The trail drops gradually as it heads towards the bottomlands of Tarkington Bayou and enters a clear-cut where young trees are beginning their lives.

▲ Campsite

At **MILE MARKER 84** reach Tarkington Bayou, which at first looks like any small seasonal creek. Here, you are within 5 miles of its headwaters. As you continue, you cross the bayou again on a hiker bridge at mile 84.3 and notice that already its waters are improving in depth and quality (as long as the season is not too dry). Cross a small dirt road at mile 84.8 and enter mature woodland where a prescribed burn was set in early 2006. Pass **MILE MARKERS 85** and **86** as the trail meanders alongside the bayou, which remains on your left. (Remember that if you are westbound, you need to reverse all directions, left and right, in these trail descriptions.)

Just after mile 86, follow a small logging road for a short distance before turning right (do not cross the Tarkington Bayou here). In some years, the bayou's waters may recede underground for a while, leaving the hiker without a water supply, save for some old murky oxbows, like the one at mile 86.6. Pass **MILE MARKER 87** next to the creek. Even if the bayou is dry here, it continues to be an easy, picturesque walk through a mature pine-dominated forest. You veer away from the bayou for good by mile 87.3.

Just after **MILE MARKER 88**, cross a pipeline right-of-way and continue ahead on a straight path through a young pine forest that is open enough to allow

Campsite ▲ waterless camping. ▲ Cross a seasonal drainage at mile 88.5 and a faint logging road at mile 88.7. Soon after, walk near an old fence line and its adjacent old road. At mile 88.9, take a left onto a logging road and pass **MILE MARKER 89**. Watch for the sharp right turn at mile 89.1; the trail still appears to follow the logging road. The forest has grown more mature with thick scrub brush as undergrowth. You may be able to spot more longleaf pines in this area. Cross a hiker bridge at a seasonal wetland and creek where a farmstead is visible off to the left. At mile 89.8, the trail crosses a red dirt road near private property. Dogs may bark at you here.

Around **MILE MARKER 90**, cross a series of abandoned jeep tracks, one of which you follow. At least one of these junctions can be confusing if you are walking eastbound since there are few trail markers; at the junction, veer slightly to the right (don't take a hard right) and then stay straight. At mile 90.1, in a mix of trees, including holly and magnolia, there is a small clearing **Campsite** ▲ for one waterless campsite. ▲ FM 2025, which runs north-south, is reached at mile 90.7. (The LSHT here has turned westward briefly.) LSHT Trailhead Parking Lot #14 is located along FM 2025 (thru-hikers may be interested to know that a gas station with a convenience store is located about 1 mile to the (left) south at the junction of FM 2025 and FM 945).

The LSHT reenters the woods directly across the paved road. At mile 90.8, cross a seasonal drainage. Enter a hardwood forest dominated by white oak and hickory. A few open areas under pines present **Campsite** ▲ themselves as potential waterless campsites ▲ just before **MILE MARKER 91**. Parallel a seasonal drainage on the right and then cross a small creek that may harbor water at mile 91.2. Between miles 91.4 and 91.5, follow an old railroad bed. In the next half mile, you pass many water oaks and swamp chestnut oaks, both water-tolerant oak species. Reach a small creek that normally has good water in it at mile 91.8. You may have to hop over this creek, or cross on a downed log, if it is running hard. The palmetto bottomlands through here flood regularly, so be prepared to wade through ankle-deep water if the season has been wet.

Pass **MILE MARKER 92**, followed by a seasonal creek at mile 92.3. Just after this creek, you should spot the muddy waters of the East Fork of the San Jacinto River on the right. The river is quickly crossed on a large steel hiker bridge at mile 92.4. Follow a dirt road straight ahead, watching for the trail to head off into the woods to the left within 0.1 mile. It would be difficult and potentially dangerous to scramble down the banks of the river here to get water; be very cautious and consider other water sources instead.

Pass through a wetland area where buttonbush (a shrub with greenish white flowers) and blue waterleaf (a deep blue flower with five petals) bloom in the spring. In a young pine forest, cross an often stagnant creek at mile 92.5. The trail is open and pleasant in this area, but expect some large standing puddles in wet seasons. At mile 92.8, cross a small hiker bridge over a wetland. Reach Highway 945 and cross it on a diagonal to the right. There is no official trail parking here (however, thru-hikers may be interested to know that there is a combination gas station and convenience store 1.4 miles away at the intersection of Highway 945 and FM 2025; eastbounders turn left, east, on FM 945 to reach the store).

Very soon after, reach **MILE MARKER 93** and cross a fence line (you may notice another number, such as 18 in this case, on the mile markers between the eastern terminus and Double Lake; this number represents the miles westbound back to Double Lake). At mile 93.2, you may notice the concrete pillars of an old lookout tower's base. Another fire tower base is located at mile 93.8 adjacent to a creek that usually has clear, running water in it. Take a sharp right on an old road, walk a little way down it, and then take a hard left (the road continues straight ahead, so be careful not to stay on it). The trail may be wet in this area, even though it now follows another old roadbed. Pass **MILE MARKER 94** and yet another fire tower base.

Cross well-maintained gravel Forest Service Road 274A at mile 94.4. These forests are comprised of mostly hardwoods; the wet soil also lends itself to the growth of ferns, vines, and dwarf palmettos. Hikers who have a good eye may spot the elusive Louisiana palm (*Sabal louisiana*),which has been sighted near the LSHT in this area. Though the Louisiana palm does grow in the San Jacinto River bottomlands near Cleveland, it is not common in Texas. Often confused with the dwarf palmetto when it is young, the Louisiana palm can grow as tall as 18 feet (though it is usually 3 to 6 feet tall) with a trunk 2 feet in diameter. The common dwarf palmetto is also considered a palm, but does not have a trunk.

At mile 94.8, cross a gravel road followed by a hiker bridge over a seasonal creek. Sadly, this road leads to an oil and gas well drilled in the heart of Winters Bayou Scenic Area. A long boardwalk now takes you through a palmetto swamp, which may distract you from noticing **MILE MARKER 95**. Farther on, another bridge helps keep your feet dry over a wetland. These are the bottomlands of Winters Bayou, another large creek that joins up with the East Fork of the San Jacinto about 3 miles downstream from here. Reach the banks of Winters Bayou at mile 95.4, crossing it on another large steel bridge soon after. At mile 95.6, cross a

An unusually tall Southern magnolia towers over the LSHT near the eastern terminus.

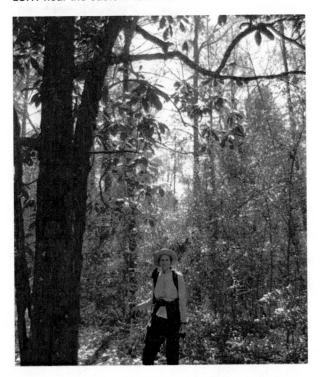

shallow bayou on a bridge, under overhead phone lines and over another bridged wetland. One final bridge leads over a wet area at mile 95.8. Now the trail takes you through an old clear-cut and past **MILE MARKER 96** before meeting up with older forest. Very large Southern magnolias and white oaks grow here.

Once you spot the white church and barbed wire fence, you're at the end of the LSHT. The Winters Bayou lot, LSHT Trailhead Parking Lot #15, is a large gravel area off of FM 1725. This is the eastern terminus of the Lone Star Hiking Trail. Congratulations, eastbound thru-hikers!

SECTION 10 MILEAGE

MILES W→E	TRAIL POINT	MILES E→W	NOTES
82.3	LSHT Trailhead Parking Lot #13; FM 2666	13.8	⚊ 🅿
82.6	Hiker gate	13.5	
83.0	**MILE MARKER 83**	13.1	
83.2	Corner benchmark and bearing tree; ATV/horse track	12.9	
83.3	Primitive campsite	12.8	▲
83.4	Bridge over creek (stagnant water)	12.7	🚰 *
83.7	Seasonal drainage	12.4	
84.0	**MILE MARKER 84; reach Tarkington Bayou**	12.1	🚰 *
84.3	Hiker bridge over Tarkington Bayou (dark, clear water)	11.8	🚰
84.8	Jeep road	11.3	
85.0	**MILE MARKER 85**	10.1	
86.0	Logging road; **MILE MARKER 86;** follow LSHT left, then right	9.5	
86.6	Oxbow pond of Tarkington Bayou (muddy)	9.1	🚰
87.0	**MILE MARKER 87;** veer away from Tarkington Bayou for good	8.1	
88.0	**MILE MARKER 88**	8.0	
88.1	Pipeline right-of-way; potential camping	7.6	▲
88.5	Seasonal drainage	7.4	
88.7	Old logging track	7.3	
88.8	Old fence line and adjacent road	7.2	
88.9	Turn left on logging road	7.1	
89.0	**MILE MARKER 89**	7.0	
89.1	Sharp turn to right	6.5	
89.6	Bridge over creek (stagnant water); farmstead on left	6.3	🚰 *
89.8	Red dirt road near private homes	6.1	⚊
90.0	**MILE MARKER 90;** abandoned jeep roads; confusing junction; follow LSHT slightly to right and then straight	6.0	
90.1	Potential waterless campsite	5.9	▲
90.7	FM 2025; LSHT Trailhead Parking Lot #14 (store 1 mile south)	5.4	⚊ 🅿
90.8	Seasonal drainage	5.3	
91.0	Potential campsites; **MILE MARKER 91**	5.1	▲
91.2	Cross at a junction of small creeks (low flow; clear water)	4.9	🚰 *

SECTION 10 MILEAGE

MILES W→E	TRAIL POINT	MILES E→W	NOTES
91.4	Left turn onto old railroad bed	4.7	
91.8	Unbridged seasonal creek (strong flow; clear water)	4.3	🚰
92.0	**MILE MARKER 92;** creek on right (stagnant water)	4.1	
92.3	Seasonal creek; East Fork of San Jacinto River on right	3.8	🚰
92.4	Steel hiker bridge over East Fork of San Jacinto River (deep, muddy water)	3.7	🚰
92.5	Seasonal creek (stagnant water)	3.6	
92.8	Bridge over wetland	3.3	
93.0	Highway 945 (combination gas station and store 1.4 miles east); **MILE MARKER 93**	3.1	▬
93.2	Old fire tower base	2.9	
93.8	Creek (clear water; good flow); old fire tower base	2.3	🚰
94.0	Sharp right on old road, then sharp left to leave road; **MILE MARKER 94** a little beyond (last "mile" was 1.2 miles long)	2.1	
94.1	Old fire tower base	2.0	
94.4	Gravel road FS 274A	1.7	
94.8	Pipeline with road; hiker bridge over seasonal creek	1.3	
95.0	**MILE MARKER 95**	1.1	
95.4	Steel hiker bridge over Winters Bayou (deep, muddy water)	0.7	🚰
95.7	Phone lines; boardwalk over wet area	0.4	
96.0	**MILE MARKER 96**	0.1	
96.1	LSHT Trailhead Parking Lot #15; FM 1725; eastern terminus of LSHT	0.0	▬ 🅿

* *Water here is seasonal and dependent on weather conditions.*

MILEAGE CHART KEY

🚰	Water source	▲	Undeveloped campsite or potential camping area
🚐	Developed campground		
🅿	Parking area/trailhead	▬▬▬	Major roads (jeep tracks and logging roads are not indicated)

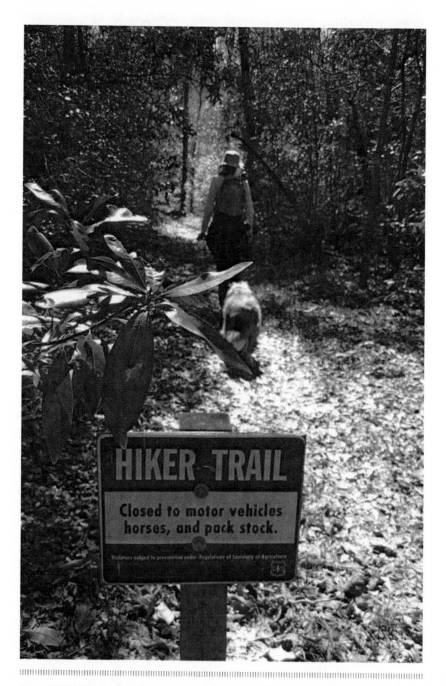

A peaceful afternoon afoot on the LSHT in the Bayou Section

Appendixes

APPENDIX A

RESOURCES AND CONTACT INFORMATION

Be aware that cell phone service along many parts of the LSHT is not reliable because of the trail's remote character.

Double Lake Recreation Area
www.fs.fed.us/r8/texas/recreation/sam_houston/doublelake.shtml

Houston Regional Group of the Sierra Club
P.O. Box 3021
Houston, TX 77253
(713) 895-9309
http://houston.sierraclub.org

Huntsville State Park
P.O. Box 508
Huntsville, TX 77342
(936) 295-5644
www.tpwd.state.tx.us/spdest/findadest/parks/huntsville

Lone Star Hiking Trail Club, Inc.
113 Ben Drive
Houston, TX 77022
www.lshtclub.com

National Forest Maps
U.S. Department of Agriculture, Forest Service
415 South First Street, Suite 110
Lufkin, TX 75901
www.fs.fed.us/r8/texas/maps/

Sam Houston National Forest
394 FM 1375 West
New Waverly, TX 77358
(936) 344-6205, ext. 221; toll free (888) 361-6908
Office hours: 8:00 AM–4:30 PM Monday–Friday
www.fs.fed.us/r8/texas/recreation/sam_houston/samhouston_rec_opps.shtml

USGS Quads / Topographic Maps:
store.usgs.gov
www.terraserver-usa.com

EMERGENCIES	
24-hour emergency	911
Sam Houston Ranger District	(936) 344-6205
Huntsville Police Department	(936) 435-8001
Liberty County Sheriff's Office	(281) 592-3411
Montgomery County Sheriff's Office	(936) 760-5800
San Jacinto County Sheriff's Office	(936) 653-4367
Walker County Sheriff's Office	(936) 435-8001
Conroe Regional Medical Center	(936) 539-1111
Cleveland Regional Medical Center	(281) 593-1811
Huntsville Memorial Hospital	(936) 291-3411

APPENDIX B

REFERENCES AND RECOMMENDED READING

Ajilvsgi, Geyata. *Wildflowers of Texas*. Fredericksburg, Tex.: Shearer Publishing, 1984.

Covey, Cyclone. *Adventures in the Unknown Interior of America by Cabeza de Vaca*. Albuquerque: University of New Mexico Press, 1993.

Fletcher, Colin, and Chip Rawlins. *The Complete Walker IV*. New York City: Knopf, 2002.

The Heritage of North Harris County. North Harris County Branch: American Association of University Women, 1977.

Rappole, John H., and Gene W. Blacklock. *Birds of Texas*. Houston: Rice University Press, 1990.

Robison, B. C. *Birds of Houston*. Houston: Rice University Press, 1990.

Schimelpfenig, Todd, Linda Lindsey, and Joan Safford. *NOLS Wilderness First Aid*. Mechanicsburg, Penn.: Stackpole Books, 2000.

Tull, Delena, and George Oxford Miller. *Lone Star Field Guide to Wildflowers, Trees, and Shrubs of Texas*. Houston: Gulf Publishing Company, 1991.

Tveten, John, and Gloria Tveten. *Wildflowers of Houston and Southeast Texas*. Austin: University of Texas Press, 1993.

Vines, Robert A. *Trees of East Texas*. Austin: University of Texas Press, 1977.

Watson, Geraldine Ellis. *Big Thicket Plant Ecology*. Denton: University of North Texas Press, 2006.

APPENDIX C

EQUIPMENT AND FOOD CHECKLISTS

Dayhiking Equipment Checklist

BASICS	CLOTHING	FIRST AID	OPTIONAL
Backpack	T-shirt	Gauze	Hiking poles
Backpack rain cover	Shorts	Band-aids	Bandanna
Water containers	Pants	Pain reliever	Gaiters
Water filter or chemical treatment	Rain jacket	Waterproof medical tape	Liner socks
Guidebook and maps	Fleece jacket	Antibiotic ointment	Watch
Compass	Warm hat or balaclava	Blister treatment	Eyeglasses
Lighter or matches	Sun hat	Lip balm	Sunglasses
Pocket knife	Gloves		Camera
Headlamp or flashlight	Socks		Binoculars
Sunscreen	Boots or hiking shoes		
Insect repellent	Insoles		
Toilet paper			
ziploc bags			

Backpacking Equipment Checklist

Note: Add these items to the above dayhiking checklist.

BASICS	CLOTHING	TOILETRIES	OPTIONAL
Tent (rain fly, tent poles, and stakes)	Extra T-shirt	Toothbrush and toothpaste	Stuff sacks (for food, clothes, etc.)
Ground cloth	Extra shorts	Dental floss	Plastic camp mirror
Sleeping bag	Extra pants	Brush or comb	Paper and pen
Sleeping pad	Long underwear	Hair tie or clip	Extra ziploc bags
Cook pot with lid	Extra underwear	Hand sanitizer	Earplugs
Cook stove with wind-screen	Camp shoes (e.g., sandals)	Feminine hygiene products	Pack towel
Fuel	Extra socks		Spare batteries
Spoon			
Duct tape			
30 feet of cord or rope			

Hiking and Backpacking Food Ideas

BREAKFAST	LUNCH	SNACKS	DINNER
Cereal	Bread products (e.g., tortillas, bagels, or pita)	Gorp (mixture of granola and dried fruits and nuts)	Prepackaged rice or noodle meals (e.g., Knorr Pasta Sides or Pasta Roni)
Dehydrated milk	Peanut butter	Nuts	Instant soups
Dried fruit	Tuna or other canned (or pouched) meat	Dried or fresh fruit	Couscous
Granola bars	Crackers	Energy bars	Dried textured vegetable protein (TVP)
Energy bars	Cheese	Cookies or snack cakes	Tuna or other canned (or pouched) meat
Peanut butter sandwich	Beef jerky	Pretzels (plain or yogurt) or chips	Instant mashed potatoes
Instant oatmeal	Summer sausage	Candy or chocolate bars	Dehydrated vegetables
Pop tarts		Hot cocoa, tea, or powdered drink mixes	Olive oil (in a small plastic bottle)

APPENDIX D

Consolidated Mileage of the LSHT

Note: A 💧* indicates that water there is seasonal and dependent on weather conditions. In Section 9, LSHT mile markers 76–79 are not yet in place on rerouted trail.

MILES W→E	TRAIL POINT	MILES E→W	NOTES
★	**SECTION 1**		
0.0	Western terminus of LSHT; FS 219 at FM 149 LSHT Richards Trailhead Parking Lot #1	96.1	▬ 🅿
0.1	Little Lake Creek Loop Trail (orange-blazed) branches right; follow LSHT left	96.0	
0.2	Utilities right-of-way	95.9	
0.4	Seasonal drainage on left	95.7	
1.0	**MILE MARKER 1**; potential camping	95.1	⛺
1.3	Large seasonal drainage	94.8	
1.8	FS 2031A (good dirt road)	94.3	▬
2.0	Small seasonal drainage; **MILE MARKER 2**	94.1	
2.1	LSHT blazed in two directions; follow LSHT left parallel to FS 203 (good dirt road)	94.0	▬
2.2	Abandoned jeep road	93.9	
2.5	Small pond (semi-clear water); potential camping	93.6	💧⛺
2.7	ATV/jeep track; large seasonal drainage	93.4	
3.0	**MILE MARKER 3**	93.1	
3.3	Junction with West Fork Trail; large seasonal drainage	92.8	
3.4	FS 211 (good dirt road); LSHT Sandy Branch Trailhead Parking Lot #2; enter Little Lake Creek (LLC) Wilderness	92.7	▬ 🅿
3.7	Hiker gate at a fence	92.4	
3.8	Wilderness Trail branches left; follow LSHT straight	92.3	
4.0	**MILE MARKER 4**; creek (low volume; good water)	92.1	💧*
4.6	Large seasonal drainage (stagnant water)	91.5	
5.0	**MILE MARKER 5**	91.1	
5.1	Intersect Sand Branch Trail; follow LSHT left; LLC Wilderness boundary	91.0	

MILES W→E	TRAIL POINT	MILES E→W	NOTES
5.8	Old (inaccurate) wooden milepost "6"	90.3	
5.9	Boardwalks over Little Lake Creek bottomland	90.2	
6.0	**MILE MARKER 6**	90.1	
6.5	LLC Wilderness boundary; jeep road	89.6	
6.7	ATV track on right	89.4	
6.8	Pole Creek Trail (blue-blazed) to right; follow LSHT left	89.3	
7.0	**MILE MARKER 7**	89.1	
7.2	Creek adjacent to trail (low volume; good water)	88.9	🚰*
7.7	Hiker bridge over deep drainage	88.4	
7.9	Old wooden milepost "8"	88.2	
8.0	**MILE MARKER 8**; potential camping; creek (low volume; good water)	88.1	▲🚰
8.6	Utilities right-of-way	87.5	
8.7	FM 149; LSHT North Wilderness Trailhead Parking Lot #3	87.4	⬛ P
★	**SECTION 2**		
8.7	FM 149; LSHT North Wilderness Trailhead Parking Lot #3	87.4	⬛ P
8.9	Junction of trails; follow LSHT left	87.2	
9.0	**MILE MARKER 9**	87.1	
9.1	Jeep track; follow LSHT left	87.0	
9.3	Junction of trails; follow LSHT left	86.8	
9.8	Pond (hard to see) on left	86.3	
10.0	**MILE MARKER 10**	86.1	
10.5	Potential waterless campsites	85.6	▲
10.9	T-junction; follow LSHT right	85.2	
11.0	**MILE MARKER 11**	85.1	
11.3	Osborn Road (FS 237); trailhead parking	84.8	⬛ P
11.4	Utilities right-of-way	84.7	
11.8	Little Lake Creek Loop branches right; follow LSHT straight ahead	84.3	
11.9	Caney Creek (high volume; good water); potential camping	84.2	🚰▲
12.0	**MILE MARKER 12; swampy area**	84.1	
12.2	Large seasonal drainage	83.9	
12.7	ATV track at top of hill	83.4	
12.8	Creek (low volume; good water)	83.3	🚰*

MILES W→E	TRAIL POINT	MILES E→W	NOTES
13.0	Old wooden milepost; **MILE MARKER 13**	83.1	
13.1	Seasonal creek	83.0	
13.3	Pipeline right-of-way; gravel access road	82.8	
13.7	Creek (stagnant water)	82.4	
14.0	**MILE MARKER 14**	82.1	
14.2	ATV track	81.9	
14.4	FS 271 (good dirt road); FS 204 (paved road); Kelly's Pond Campground 1 mile right on FS 271	81.7	▭ 🏕
14.7	ATV track	81.4	
15.0	**MILE MARKER 15;** potential camping; creek (low volume; murky)	81.1	🚰 ▲
15.6	Seasonal creek	80.5	
15.8	FM 1375; LSHT Stubblefield Trailhead Parking Lot #6	80.3	▭ 🅿
★ SECTION 3			
15.8	FM 1375; LSHT Stubblefield Trailhead Parking Lot #6	80.3	▭ 🅿
16.0	**MILE MARKER 16**	80.1	
16.5	Lake Conroe shoreline; large campsite	79.6	🚰 ▲
16.8	Creek (medium volume; slow-flowing, semi-clear water)	79.3	🚰
17.0	**MILE MARKER 17**	79.1	
17.3	Potential campsite	78.8	▲
17.5	Seasonal drainage; wetlands	78.6	
17.9	Large creek (medium volume; good water)	78.2	🚰
18.0	Cross seasonal drainage; **MILE MARKER 18**	78.1	
18.3	Jeep trail; potential campsites	77.8	▲
19.0	**MILE MARKER 19**	77.1	
19.2	Swampy creek (stagnant water)	76.9	
19.7	Stubblefield Lake Campground	76.4	▭ 🚰 🅿 🏕
20.0	FS 215 road bridge; **MILE MARKER 20**	76.1	▭
20.3	End road walk and reenter woods to right of road	75.8	
21.0	**MILE MARKER 21;** unstriped, paved road; utilities right-of-way	75.1	▭
21.4	ATV track	74.7	
21.5	Potential campsites	74.6	▲
21.7	Fire break or pipeline right-of-way	74.4	

MILES W→E	TRAIL POINT	MILES E→W	NOTES
21.9	Seasonal creek	74.2	
22.0	**MILE MARKER 22;** property boundary; potential campsites	74.1	▲
22.2	Stony-bottomed seasonal creek; wooden milepost 22	73.9	
22.3	Turn right onto old jeep track	73.8	
22.6	Jeep road splits; take left fork	73.5	
23.0	Private farm on left; **MILE MARKER 23**	73.1	
23.1	FM 1374	73.0	▬
23.5	Turn left onto large dirt road for a few hundred feet	72.6	
24.0	**MILE MARKER 24**	72.1	
24.5	Turn right onto dirt road for 0.2 mile	71.6	
24.7	Turn left onto LSHT and reenter woods	71.4	
25.0	**MILE MARKER 25**	71.1	
25.2	Large seasonal drainage	70.9	
25.3	Old logging road	70.8	
26.0	Potential campsite; **MILE MARKER 26**	70.1	▲
26.1	Take a right onto jeep track	70.0	
26.4	Old metal gate; turn right onto dirt Bath Road	69.7	▬
27.0	**MILE MARKER 27** along Bath Road	69.1	
27.9	Intersection of Bath and Ball roads; turn right onto Ball Road	68.2	▬
28.0	**MILE MARKER 28** along Ball Road	68.1	
28.1	Turn left onto gravel Cotton Creek Cemetery Road	68.0	▬
28.3	National forest property boundary; swing left on old dirt road	67.7	
★	**SECTION 4**		
28.3	National forest property boundary; swing left on old dirt road	67.7	
28.4	Leave old dirt road; turn right over hump into woods on LSHT	67.7	
28.9	Pond	67.2	🚰 ▲
29.0	**MILE MARKER 29**	67.1	
29.5	Seasonal drainage; old wooden milepost 29; turn right	66.6	
30.0	Cross pipeline right-of-way; **MILE MARKER 30**	66.1	▲
30.1	Seasonal drainage	66.0	
30.2	Cross old fence line and hiker gate	65.9	
30.7	Enter open area with potential camping; seasonal drainage	65.4	▲
31.0	Seasonal drainage; **MILE MARKER 31;** large clearing	65.1	
31.3	Elkins Lake Subdivision water treatment plant visible	64.8	

MILES W→E	TRAIL POINT	MILES E→W	NOTES
31.5	Seasonal stream	64.6	
32.0	MILE MARKER 32; Elkins Lake Subdivision; turn left on paved road	64.1	☒
32.1	Cross Camelia Lake spillway	64.0	
32.6	Seasonal drainage; potential waterless campsites in pine forest	63.5	▲
33.0	MILE MARKER 33	63.1	
33.1	Cross tributary of Alligator Branch; swamps	63.0	
33.3	Alligator Branch	62.8	🚰 ▲
33.7	Old wooden milepost 33	62.4	
33.8	Cross old railroad bed	62.3	
34.0	MILE MARKER 34	62.1	
34.8	Junction of trails; turn right to follow LSHT	61.3	
35.0	MILE MARKER 35; Interstate 45; LSHT Huntsville Trailhead Parking Lot #7; turn right on I-45 feeder road	61.1	☒ 🅿
35.6	Turn left on Park Road 40 and continue under I-45 (Huntsville State Park is approximately 1 mile to the right on Park Road 40)	60.5	☒
36.0	MILE MARKER 36 on Park Road 40	60.1	
36.6	Turn right onto Highway 75	59.5	☒
36.7	Turn left onto Evelyn Lane	59.4	☒
36.9	Turn left onto LSHT right of blue metal gate in woods	59.2	
★	SECTION 5		
36.9	Turn left into woods right of blue metal gate on Evelyn Lane	59.2	☒
37.0	MILE MARKER 37	59.1	
37.4	Seasonal drainage; abandoned logging road	58.7	
37.6	Old wooden milepost 37; large sandy-bottomed gully	58.5	
37.7	Steep-sided seasonal drainage	58.4	
37.8	Jeep track	58.3	
38.0	MILE MARKER 38 in open grassy area; potential campsite	58.1	▲
38.2	Bridge over small seasonal creek (stagnant water)	57.9	
38.4	Grass-covered logging road	57.7	
38.6	Old wooden milepost 38	57.5	
38.7	Seasonal drainage	57.4	
38.9	Potential campsite under holly tree on left	57.2	▲
39.0	MILE MARKER 39	57.1	
39.1	Follow jeep track left across power line	57.0	

MILES W→E	TRAIL POINT	MILES E→W	NOTES
39.4	Hiker gate; left onto gravel road (Evelyn Lane)	56.7	▬
39.7	Reenter woods on left	56.4	
40.0	Old logging road; **MILE MARKER 40**	56.1	
40.4	Bridged seasonal creek (small amount of flowing water)	55.7	
40.5	Large seasonal creek (stagnant water)	55.6	
40.6	Seasonal creek	55.5	
41.0	**MILE MARKER 41**	55.1	
41.2	Gravel road	54.9	
41.6	Old logging road	54.5	
41.7	Seasonal drainage	54.4	
41.9	Pipeline crossing	54.2	
42.0	**MILE MARKER 42;** left onto FM 2296	54.1	▬
42.6	Right onto unstriped, paved Four Notch Road	53.5	▬
42.8	Cross railroad tracks; continue on Four Notch Road	53.3	
43.0	Creek (low volume); **MILE MARKER 43** along Four Notch Road	53.1	🚰 *
43.7	Cross Winters Bayou on Four Notch Road bridge (high volume)	52.4	🚰
44.0	**MILE MARKER 44** on Four Notch Road	52.1	
44.9	Left onto dirt FS 213	51.2	▬
45.0	**MILE MARKER 45** on FS 213	51.1	
45.1	LSHT Four Notch Trailhead Parking Lot #8; reenter woods on right	51.0	▬ 🅿
★	**SECTION 6**		
45.1	LSHT Four Notch Trailhead Parking Lot #8; reenter woods on right	51.0	▬ 🅿
45.4	Junction with Four Notch Loop Trail; main LSHT turns right	50.7	
45.7	Deep seasonal drainage; logging road	50.4	
45.9	Seasonal creek	50.2	
46.0	Faint logging road; **MILE MARKER 46**	50.1	
46.2	Seasonal creek	49.9	
46.5	Trash-filled hunter camp on dirt road; potential campsites	49.6	▲
46.7	Potential campsites on right; parallel seasonal drainage on right	49.4	▲
46.8	Large seasonal creek	49.3	
47.0	**MILE MARKER 47;** seasonal creek	49.1	
47.1	Left onto old logging road	49.0	

MILES W→E	TRAIL POINT	MILES E→W	NOTES
47.2	Cross logging road	48.9	
47.4	Large open flat; potential camping	48.7	▲
47.5	Right onto old logging road	48.6	
47.6	Large open flat; potential camping; seasonal creek	48.5	▲
47.8	Junction of old logging roads	48.3	
48.0	**MILE MARKER 48**	48.1	
48.2	Boswell Creek; camping (high volume; good water)	47.9	🚰 ▲
48.7	Seasonal drainage	47.4	
49.0	**MILE MARKER 49**	47.1	
49.4	Junction with Four Notch Loop Trail	46.7	
49.5	Small seasonal drainage; hill	46.6	
49.9	Bridge over Briar Creek (low flow; good water)	46.2	🚰
50.0	**MILE MARKER 50**	46.1	
50.4	Cross over FS 206	45.7	▭
51.0	**MILE MARKER 51; pipeline right-of-way**	45.1	
51.1	Large seasonal creek	45.0	
51.3	Large seasonal creek	44.8	
51.5	Pond on left; camping (dark tannin-colored water)	44.6	🚰 ▲
51.8	Left onto gravel FS 200	44.3	▭
51.9	Creek (low volume; good water) along FS 200	44.2	🚰
52.0	**MILE MARKER 52** (not visible on road)	44.1	
52.4	Turn right onto gravel FS 207 at stop sign	43.7	▭
53.0	Gas processing plant; **MILE MARKER 53** (not visible on road)	43.1	
54.0	**MILE MARKER 54** (not visible on road)	42.1	
54.4	Junction of FS 207 and 202; reenter woods	41.7	▭ 🅿
★	**SECTION 7**		
54.4	Junction of FS 207 and 202; reenter woods	41.7	▭ 🅿
54.6	Deep seasonal drainage; potential camping	41.5	▲
55.0	Series of seasonal drainages; **MILE MARKER 55**	41.1	
55.3	Set of twin seasonal drainages	40.8	
55.4	Cross sunken road twice; potential campsite	40.7	▲
55.8	Cross seasonal drainage twice (stagnant water)	40.3	
56.0	**MILE MARKER 56; drainage to the left crossed in 0.1 mile**	40.1	
56.2	Seasonal drainage (trickle of water) (West Fork Caney Creek)	39.9	

MILES W→E	TRAIL POINT	MILES E→W	NOTES
56.9	West Fork Caney Creek (low volume; clear); property boundary	39.2	⌀ *
57.0	MILE MARKER 57	39.1	
57.7	Shallow seasonal drainage; larger U-shaped drainage	38.4	
58.0	MILE MARKER 58; potential camping	38.1	▲
58.1	Old road bed	38.0	
58.2	Cross fern-lined seasonal drainage twice	37.9	
58.5	Logging track	37.6	
58.8	Large oak tree; potential campsites	37.3	▲
59.0	MILE MARKER 59	37.1	
59.1	Fern-lined seasonal drainage (Chinquapin Creek)	37.0	
59.5	Seasonal drainage	36.6	
59.8	Small gravel road	36.3	
60.0	MILE MARKER 60; several small drainages and old logging road	36.1	
60.2	Old jeep track heads uphill to left; follow LSHT straight ahead	35.9	
60.4	Cross large sandy-bottomed intermittent stream	35.7	
60.6	Cross several small seasonal drainages	35.5	
60.9	Junction of trails; follow LSHT left	35.2	
61.0	MILE MARKER 61	35.1	
61.4	Open area at junction of logging roads; potential camping; follow LSHT straight and then right	34.7	▲
61.5	Make a sharp left turn	34.6	
61.7	Deep brushy seasonal drainage	34.4	
62.0	MILE MARKER 62	34.1	
62.4	Fence post and corner at property boundary	33.7	
62.8	LSHT Big Woods Trailhead Parking Lot #9; follow LSHT left onto dirt Ira Denson Road	33.3	⊷ 🅿
★	SECTION 8		
62.8	LSHT Big Woods Trailhead Parking Lot #9; follow LSHT left onto dirt Ira Denson Road	33.3	⊷ 🅿
63.0	MILE MARKER 63; intersection of Ira Denson Rd. and FS 202	33.1	⊷
64.0	MILE MARKER 64	32.1	
64.7	Intersection of FS 202 (John Warren Rd.) and Hwy. 150; follow LSHT left on Hwy. 150	31.4	⊷
65.0	MILE MARKER 65; intersection of Hwy. 150 and FM 945 in Evergreen; follow LSHT right on FM 945	31.1	⊷

MILES W→E	TRAIL POINT	MILES E→W	NOTES
65.5	Cemetery on left along FM 945	30.6	
66.0	**MILE MARKER 66**	30.1	
67.0	**MILE MARKER 67**	29.1	
67.4	Intersection of FM 945 and Butch Arther Rd. (Jacobs Rd.); LSHT Trailhead Parking Lot #10	28.7	⚊ 🅿
67.9	Seasonal drainage	28.2	
68.0	**MILE MARKER 68**	28.1	
68.2	Hiker bridge over large seasonal drainage (low flow; good water)	27.9	🚰 *
68.4	Seasonal drainage	27.7	
68.6	LSHT Primitive Campsite #2 to right of trail	27.5	▲
69.0	**MILE MARKER 69**	27.1	
69.1	Fence corner	27.0	
69.2	Creek (low flow; good water)	26.9	🚰 *
69.3	Fence corner	26.8	
69.4	Creek (low flow; good water)	26.7	🚰 *
69.8	ATV track; horse farm	26.3	
69.9	Dirt road	26.2	
70.0	**MILE MARKER 70**	26.1	
70.1	Hiker bridge over drainage (low flow; good water)	26.0	🚰 *
70.6	Hiker gate; stay straight	25.5	
71.0	**MILE MARKER 71; intersect orange-striped trail; follow LSHT straight**	25.1	
71.1	Bridge over East Fork San Jacinto River	25.0	🚰
71.3	Hiker bridge over creek (deep, clear water)	24.8	🚰
71.7	Hiker bridge over stream (shallow, clear water)	24.4	🚰 *
72.0	**MILE MARKER 72; pipeline right-of-way; gravel jeep track**	24.1	
72.2	Hiker bridge over creek (shallow, clear water)	23.9	🚰 *
72.3	Potential campsite on left	23.8	▲
72.4	Gravel road; utilities right-of-way	23.7	
72.6	Old logging road; clearing to the right	23.5	
72.8	Old roadbed; make sharp right turn and follow old road	23.3	
72.9	Metal gate; logging road	23.2	
73.0	**MILE MARKER 73**	23.1	
73.1	Sharp right turn; hiker bridge over seasonal drainage	23.0	
73.7	FM 2025; LSHT Trailhead Parking Lot #11	22.4	⚊ 🅿

MILES W→E	TRAIL POINT	MILES E→W	NOTES
73.8	Potential camping (close to road); utility lines	22.3	▲
73.9	Two hiker gates	22.2	
74.0	**MILE MARKER 74**	22.1	
74.8	Open area; reach gravel nature trail on top of old railroad bed; potential camping	21.3	▲
74.9	Old road	21.2	
75.0	Double Lake Recreation Area; **MILE MARKER 75**	21.1	🚰 ⛲ 🅿 🍽
★	**SECTION 9**		
75.0	Double Lake Recreation Area; **MILE MARKER 75**	21.1	🚰 ⛲ 🅿 🍽
75.1	Utilities right-of-way; intersect mountain biking trail	21.0	
75.6	Gravel FS 220; hiker gate; Big Creek tributary on left	20.5	🚰 ⛲
75.7	Hiker bridge over seasonal drainage; LSHT Primitive Campsite #1; begin marked trail reroute on higher ground above creek	20.4	▲
76.0	Small bridge over deep drainage; potential camping; creek on left (good water; low flow); **MILE MARKER 76**	20.1	⛲ ▲
76.5	Small bridge over deep drainage	19.6	
76.6	Long bridge over creek; follow LSHT right	19.5	
76.9	Two bridges over small creeks (low flow; good water)	19.2	⛲
77.0	**MILE MARKER 77**	19.1	
77.6	Cross swampy creek (stagnant water)	18.5	
78.0	**MILE MARKER 78**	18.1	
78.6	Cross old railroad bed; veer left to follow LSHT through hiker gate	17.5	
79.0	**MILE MARKER 79**	17.1	
79.2	Intersect orange-blazed Big Creek Trail; follow LSHT left	16.9	
79.3	**ORIGINAL MILE MARKER 79;** intersect green-blazed White Oak Trail; follow LSHT left	16.8	
79.4	Bridge over Big Creek; intersect permanently closed, blue-blazed Magnolia Loop Trail; follow LSHT right	16.7	⛲
79.7	Long bridge over Big Creek; intersect yellow-blazed Pine Trail; follow LSHT left	16.4	⛲
79.8	Hiker bridge; intersect trail heading down to left; follow LSHT's sharp right turn	16.3	

MILES W→E	TRAIL POINT	MILES E→W	NOTES
79.9	Big Creek Scenic Area sign; short side trail to left leads to LSHT Trailhead Parking Lot #12; intersect yellow-blazed Pine Trail and orange-blazed Big Creek Trail on right; follow LSHT straight ahead on old railroad bed	16.2	🅿
80.0	MILE MARKER 80 (this "mile" is 1.3 miles long due to reroute)	16.1	
80.6	Hiker gate; gravel FS 221	15.5	▭
81.0	Small seasonal drainage; MILE MARKER 81	15.1	
81.2	Intersect unidentified trail; follow LSHT left; potential campsite; seasonal drainage	14.9	▲
82.0	MILE MARKER 82	14.1	
82.3	LSHT Tarkington Trailhead Parking Lot #13; FM 2666	13.8	▭ 🅿
★	**SECTION 10**		
82.3	LSHT Tarkington Trailhead Parking Lot #13; FM 2666	13.8	▭ 🅿
82.6	Hiker gate	13.5	
83.0	MILE MARKER 83	13.1	
83.2	Corner benchmark and bearing tree; ATV/horse track	12.9	
83.3	Primitive campsite	12.8	▲
83.4	Bridge over creek (stagnant water)	12.7	⛲ *
83.7	Seasonal drainage	12.4	
84.0	MILE MARKER 84; reach Tarkington Bayou	12.1	⛲ *
84.3	Hiker bridge over Tarkington Bayou (dark, clear water)	11.8	⛲
84.8	Jeep road	11.3	
85.0	MILE MARKER 85	10.1	
86.0	Logging road; MILE MARKER 86; follow LSHT left, then right	9.5	
86.6	Oxbow pond of Tarkington Bayou (muddy)	9.1	⛲
87.0	MILE MARKER 87; veer away from Tarkington Bayou for good	8.1	
88.0	MILE MARKER 88	8.0	
88.1	Pipeline right-of-way; potential camping	7.6	▲
88.5	Seasonal drainage	7.4	
88.7	Old logging track	7.3	
88.8	Old fence line and adjacent road	7.2	
88.9	Turn left on logging road	7.1	
89.0	MILE MARKER 89	7.0	

MILES W→E	TRAIL POINT	MILES E→W	NOTES
89.1	Sharp turn to right	6.5	
89.6	Bridge over creek (stagnant water); farmstead on left	6.3	⌁ *
89.8	Red dirt road near private homes	6.1	⚊
90.0	**MILE MARKER 90;** abandoned jeep roads; confusing junction; follow LSHT slightly to right and then straight	6.0	
90.1	Potential waterless campsite	5.9	▲
90.7	FM 2025; LSHT Trailhead Parking Lot #14 (store 1 mile south)	5.4	⚊ 🅿
90.8	Seasonal drainage	5.3	
91.0	Potential campsites; **MILE MARKER 91**	5.1	▲
91.2	Cross at a junction of small creeks (low flow; clear water)	4.9	⌁ *
91.4	Left turn onto old railroad bed	4.7	
91.8	Unbridged seasonal creek (strong flow; clear water)	4.3	⌁
92.0	**MILE MARKER 92;** creek on right (stagnant water)	4.1	
92.3	Seasonal creek; East Fork of San Jacinto River on right	3.8	⌁
92.4	Steel hiker bridge over East Fork of San Jacinto River (deep, muddy water)	3.7	⌁
92.5	Seasonal creek (stagnant water)	3.6	
92.8	Bridge over wetland	3.3	
93.0	Highway 945 (combination gas station and store 1.4 miles east); **MILE MARKER 93**	3.1	⚊
93.2	Old fire tower base	2.9	
93.8	Creek (clear water; good flow); old fire tower base	2.3	⌁
94.0	Sharp right on old road, then sharp left to leave road; **MILE MARKER 94** a little beyond (last "mile" was 1.2 miles long)	2.1	
94.1	Old fire tower base	2.0	
94.4	Gravel road FS 274A	1.7	
94.8	Pipeline with road; hiker bridge over seasonal creek	1.3	
95.0	**MILE MARKER 95**	1.1	
95.4	Steel hiker bridge over Winters Bayou (deep, muddy water)	0.7	⌁
95.7	Phone lines; boardwalk over wet area	0.4	
96.0	**MILE MARKER 96**	0.1	
96.1	LSHT Trailhead Parking Lot #15; FM 1725; eastern terminus of LSHT	0.0	⚊ 🅿

Acknowledgments

‖‖‖

during my thru-hike of the Lone Star Hiking Trail (LSHT) as I collected data for this guidebook, I had the assistance and good company of Debbie Richardson. She helped me push the measuring wheel and kept me honest regarding "right" and "left." My father, James Borski, drove us to and from the trail on several occasions and provided a comfortable base of operations. Brandt Mannchen of the Lone Star Chapter of the Sierra Club and Bill Anderson of the U.S. Forest Service were generous with their time and information about the trail and its history. Jeff Borski, Andy Somers, James Borski, Linda Woolf, June Aaron, Roslyn Bullas, Laura Shauger, and Brandt Mannchen provided much-needed advice and assistance with editing all phases of the book. Finally, I would never have followed my calling to further explore and document the LSHT without the steady encouragement and support of my partner on trails and in life, Andy Somers. Andy also created all of the maps in this guidebook—an enormous undertaking.

I must also express personal gratitude to the many volunteers who built and maintain the LSHT. Without them the trail would not exist. A portion of the proceeds gained from the sale of this book will be donated to the Lone Star Hiking Trail Club, an organization that protects and promotes the trail.

Index

About the Author

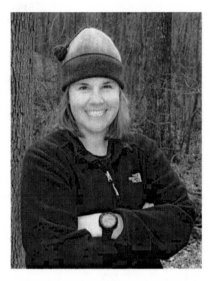

Karen Borski Somers is a native of Spring, Texas. Karen studied biomedical engineering at Texas A&M University and has spent most of her career working for NASA contractors in Clear Lake, Texas, and Huntsville, Alabama. In 1998, she thru-hiked the 2,165-mile Appalachian Trail solo and, in 2004, she hiked the 2,650-mile Pacific Crest Trail with her husband, Andy. Karen's trail name is "Nocona," a Comanche word meaning "the wanderer." She has hiked and backpacked in 36 U.S. states, logging more than 9,000 trail miles. She also bicycled 4,400 miles across the U.S. from the Atlantic to the Pacific on the TransAmerica route in 2005. Karen currently resides with her husband, daughter, and their hiking sheltie in northern Alabama. They continue their quest to summit the U.S. high points, plan expedition canoe trips, and wander on and off trails.

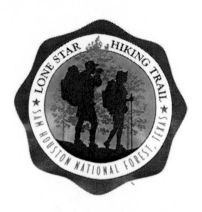

The Lone Star Hiking Trail Club

t**he Lone Star Hiking Trail Club, Inc.** was formed in 1995 on National Trails Day and is affiliated with the American Hiking Society. The club's mission is (1) to educate the public about the location, use, and needs of the hiking trails of Texas, with emphasis on the Lone Star Hiking Trail, and (2) to provide volunteer assistance for maintenance and improvement of hiking trails. Membership is open to anyone, and dues are $15 per year.

The Lone Star Hiking Trail Club counts on the support of volunteers, who are critical to the continued protection of the LSHT and perform the majority of labor required to keep the trail clear of brush, well-signed, and in good repair. Along with the Houston Regional Group of the Sierra Club, the LSHT Club acts as a watchdog, reporting to the U.S. Forest Service on trail usage statistics and conditions, as well as attending public meetings where the trail's continued status as a protected footpath is sometimes threatened.

If you spend time on the LSHT, or are planning on outing on the trail, consider joining the LSHT Club. It's a wonderful way to meet other hikers, gather information about the trail, and help protect and maintain the only long-distance footpath in Texas. Club members regularly meet on the trail for scheduled group hikes and maintenance activities. The LSHT Club also promotes camaraderie and posts information through an e-mail group.

More information is available at their website, **www.lshtclub.com,** or by writing to them at: Lone Star Hiking Trail Club, Inc., 113 Ben Drive, Houston, TX 77022.